# Statistics
# by
# Prescription

Irena Roterman-Konieczna

# Statistics by Prescription

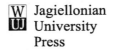 Jagiellonian University Press

This volume was supported by the Jagiellonian University – Collegium Medicum

REVIEWER
*Prof. dr hab. Andrzej Leś*

COVER DESIGN
*Marcin Bruchnalski*

ISBN 978-83-233-2741-7

www.wuj.pl

Wydawnictwo Uniwersytetu Jagiellońskiego
Redakcja: ul. Michałowskiego 9/2, 31-126 Kraków
tel. 012-631-18-81, tel./fax 012-631-18-83
Dystrybucja: ul. Wrocławska 53, 30-011 Kraków
tel. 012-631-01-97, tel./fax 012-631-01-98
tel. kom. 0506-006-674, e-mail: sprzedaz@wuj.pl
Konto: PEKAO SA, nr 80 1240 4722 1111 0000 4856 3325

*I was taught by many teachers. One of them was the MASTER:*
*Wojciech Komusiński – professor of mathematics*
*at Bartłomiej Nowodworski I-st Liceum in Kraków.*

*This book is dedicated to Him.*

# INTRODUCTION

This book is based on a series of lectures on **statistical methods delivered at the Faculty of Medicine of the Jagiellonian University Medical College**. The goal of this course is to introduce basic statistical concepts and tools necessary to analyse medical data. It is not assumed that a medical student – the future doctor – will go into raptures over statistical methods, quit his/her beautiful profession and become a statistician. It is, however, assumed that in the future professional career they both will find their common language. The doctor will communicate with the statistician and actively participate in analysis of medical data which gradually accumulate in his/her data base. If there are 10–20 patients, the doctor remembers all of them and their related events. However, when the number of patients reaches a number of thousand or even more, data analysis can be performed only with the use of statistical tools.

Trends in the development of medicine demonstrate the increasing role of monitoring and continuous analysis of medical data. The need for permanent analysis is forced by constant changes in life conditions within a given region (climate changes, wealth, fashion, lifestyle, travelling, etc.). It becomes not only necessary but also convenient to record problems the patients discuss with their doctors (family physician, hospital doctor, emergency doctor, etc.). A large number of new drugs that appear on the market also prompt individual analysis of their effects.

> The presentation of basic statistical notions and concepts is supported by examples of statistical tests performed using the SAS software package (version 3). It is assumed that the reader is familiar with Microsoft Office Excel. These statistical tests in SAS are presented in a separate section not to interrupt the continuity of statistical reasoning with technical details related to performance of a test.

The book contains also **a data base of patients admitted to the Casualty and Emergency Ward (victims of traffic accidents)**. After studying the contents of this section it is recommended to perform a series of exercises on an individual basis. References to the data base are included in sets of exercises at the end of each chapter.

> Complementary reading:
> Wayne W. Daniel: Biostatistics, John Wiley & Sons New York, Chichester, Weinheim, Brisbane, Singapore, Toronto, Seventh Edition, 1999.

(Despite its volume – which may be slightly discouraging – the book is written in a clear and concise manner. The fact that the book has seven editions indicates its popularity[1]).

Klaus Hinkelmann and Oscar Kempthorne: Design and Analysis of Experiments, Wiley, New York, Revised Edition, 1994.

Douglas C. Montgomery: Design and Analysis of Experiments, Wiley, New York, Fourth Edition, 1997.

Jerome L. Myers and Arnold D. Well: Research Design and Statistical Analysis, Earlbaum Associates, Hillsdale, NJ 1995.

---

[1] The book includes computer printouts obtained by use of the SAS software package in its older version.

# STEP 1

# Descriptive statistics – What we can learn about the patients?

Σ
Summary
Statistics

| How to find an answer to the question:
| Is it possible to avoid urolithiasis?

- **Medical problem**

It all begins with the definition of a problem; when solved, it will make doctor's work easier or when made public, it will help define risks, raise awareness and introduce preventive measures with patients, thus including also potential patients.

The definition of the medical problem is a prerequisite for successful completion of data analysis.

**To define the problem means to pose a question to which a doctor expects to get an answer after making a statistical analysis.**

Let's illustrate this with an example. A comprehensive analysis of a particular problem may serve as a model of statistical calculations in medicine. The problem to be discussed in this book is well-known to specialists. It is not our intention to provide medical instructions but the obviousness and simplicity of the medical problem will help the reader to focus on statistical methods and not medical procedures.

Our problem has been defined as **urolithiasis**. Stones in the urinary system are relatively frequent and cause major physical discomfort. One of the symptoms is acute pain (it is probably the worst pain, stronger than toothache), caused by traveling stones (crystals). In most cases, the traveling crystal resembles a spiny starfish. Sharp edges of the crystals may damage the kidney, ureter and bladder walls. The duration and severity of pain depend on stone location and its size. The presence of stones accompanied by urinary tract infection (bacterial infection) places the patient at high risk for complications. It is important to analyze what preventive measures can be applied to reduce the development of this serious and painful illness.

The human population can be divided into two subgroups: with high and low stone-forming risk. Various forms of treatment are available that can be tailored to patient's needs and specific clinical manifestations. It is beneficial for the patient to avoid acute pain and surgical intervention (those who have experienced an episode of renal colic know best). For this reason prevention is important.

By performing statistical analysis on the data pertaining to patients with urolithiasis we shall try to answer the following questions:

> **Is it possible to reduce morbidity due to urolithiasis?**
> **If so, how to reach it?**
>
> **Is it possible to avoid urolithiasis?**
> **If so, how to reach it?**

- **Data collection**

Each statistical analysis is preceded by the collection of appropriate data. Our problem has been defined as the presence of urinary stones causing painful and distressing symptoms.

Our *population*, which is subject to analysis, consists of all people who suffered from renal colic in the past, who currently have the symptoms and those who will have the illness in future.

> **A population** is a set of all the elements fulfilling specific criteria.

It is obvious that the term population is rather theoretical because in fact we shall not study *all* patients with renal colic. However, this definition limits the area of our interest excluding from analysis for instance laboratory animals that may be subject to experiments related to this illness. The fact that the number of entities belonging to this population is infinite underlines its theoretical character.

Statistical analysis, however, must be performed on concrete data pertaining to a specific group of subjects. Statistical analysis is performed on a *sample*.

> **A sample** is a subset of a population.

A sample has its size (number of elements), and it has to be representative. The purpose of our analysis is to draw conclusions from a large number of detailed data about the sampled participants that can be generalized to the population as a whole, also to those who do not belong to the primary sample. So, if we find regularity in the phenomena, we would like to generalize it to subjects who do not belong to our sample so that the conclusions from our analysis can be applied to a future patient.

> The **sample's representativeness** is determined first of all by its size and accuracy expected from our sample.

The exact formula to be followed in order to calculate the minimum group size that ensures its representativeness will be given later in this manual (after certain notions be clarified to facilitate understanding the definitions given).

A sample can be a group of people chosen at random from patients of several urological hospitals. The sample can also be constituted by all the simultaneously accessible patients from the same hospital, e.g. the one we work in. It is the second case that is going to be discussed in this handbook.

> **NOTA BENE**
> **It is essential to differentiate the population description and the sample**. This is going to be expressed in the later part of the manual by a relevant and uniform notation. Greek alphabet symbols that appear in the formula notation will refer to the population description. The given formulae using those symbols express rather the theoretical definitions of the relevant parameters (the number of elements from the population is unknown).
> Latin alphabet symbols refer to expressing the formulae with which the value of an adequate parameter for the sample can be calculated (while the sample is a set with a definite number of elements).

The notions of population and sample are accompanied by one notion of considerable importance, *number the degrees of freedom.*

Let us imagine a population of those who suffer from nephrolithiasis. Anybody asked of those produces a completely different image. It signifies that the number of degrees of freedom at the moment of the imagination was unlimited. However, if the imagination gets limited by for example the average age of patients, their gender and other parameters, the freedom for imagination gets considerably limited again step--wise depending on parameters, which make the sample more and more concrete.

> Speaking the statistics language, the **number of degrees of freedom** is gradually diminished with each respective sample definition parameter.

Defining the professional profiles, accompanying illnesses, family conditioning (congenital anatomical defects) may focus our imagination on one common sample of specific group of people.

> Generally speaking, if all the parameters concerning the group of people are given, the number of degrees of freedom may prove to be zero.

From the statistics point of view, such a situation is unfavourable, as the point of statistical analysis is to reveal certain regularities and mutual relations observed in the given group of people and the possibility to generalize them to the whole population of those who meet the condition given (i.e. the nephrolithiasis ailment). If it proves that we are working in the conditions of zero degrees of freedom, it will signify that the identified rules or relations in the given group apply only to this group.

> The larger the number of degrees of freedom in the description of a given group, the higher chances we have to generalize the obtained results to a larger community.

The above explanation is rather of an intuitive character. Mathematics introduces precisely defined ways to determine the number of degrees of freedom in any conditions.

> The number of freedom degrees is directly proportional to the number of people in the analysed sample. Hence, the larger the number of analysed elements, the larger the number of freedom degrees, and the higher the opportunity to enable the generalization of the results obtained.

Generally speaking, **the number of degrees of freedom** is expressed with the number of elements in the sample reduced by the number of already appointed parameters (mean, variance, etc.).

Each procedure of statistical concluding shows the way of appointing the freedom degrees number.[2]

- **Information record**

It is very important to determine precisely which information is essential from the point of view of the analysed question. It is also important to determine the form in which the information should be recorded and that the information coming even from several considerably different source (hospitals in Poland) is recorded in a unified and settled way. For that purpose, we determine the so-called *information record*.

The **information record** is a **complete set of organized features** that we decided to consider in our investigation.

Both these properties and the definition of measuring units (e.g. the units expressing the concentration of analysed substances in body fluids) constitute a common matrix,

---

[2] Drawing (random choice of people for analysis) is a very important stage of statistical examination, although its importance has slightly dropped in the age of information technology. Frequently the data bases are very large and their analysis is permanent.

according to which specific information that comes from each patient within the sample will be collected.

- **How to construct a correct record of information?**

It is essential that the information that constitutes certain blocks of our general issue is reasonably balanced. The point is that in case of searching for the causes of a certain phenomenon, the results were described with comparable accuracy. For example, it is unacceptable to gather a large amount of detailed information about the causes of renal colic case and describe their result with very limited number of information describing the patients condition suffering the pain. The symptoms should be described as precisely as possible. The precision of the description of the illness symptoms should be comparable with the precision of the assumed source of the illness.

> In our issue such thematic blocks can constitute the following sections: the patient's environment (e.g. family conditioning, occupation, dietary customs), the illness fit description (e.g. the painful area determining, temperature), the clinical analysis (urine composition, temperature, etc.), the therapy applied (surgical, pharmacological), the patient's condition after the therapy (complete relief, partial alleviation, etc.).[3]

Having defined the factual content of the information record, the form of presenting the specific feature should be determined. Before the record form is selected, it must be decided what kind of feature the given information item is. There is information that expresses the measure of things, and there is information that only describes a certain feature.

*Measurable features* (each feature that we describe giving the numerical value that expresses the measure of anything, e.g. the concentration of body fluids components) that present the result of the given clinical parameter measuring are no problem, as they usually are the numerical values obtained from the analytical apparatus. **The measurable features are usually put into the record and the measurement results are given**. It is important to set the measurement unit for each measurable feature.

The problem is the way of recording the information that concerns the qualitative description (like the colour of urine: straw-coloured, celadon, brown), which qualitatively only describes a given property. A letter code can be introduced then (like for determining the gender: F – feminine, M – masculine). A problem can appear when in the specific information item record a longer commentary is needed or one can expect differentiated answers. An example of such an answer in the form of a commentary can be defining the patient's occupation. We can insert the names of the jobs, e.g. bricklayer, teacher, postman, etc. Mind that sometimes those are rather long words and writing their complete forms may be hard. Moreover, errors are possible, (so that one can

---

[3] The therapeutic issues are beyond the scope of the example presented. The analysis objective is determining the prevention possibilities, hence the absence of therapy issues from this work.

write e.g. "posman"). If the profession name is accidentally misspelled, such a person will not be enumerated in the right professional group and a new category, e.g. "posman" will be created. In order to avoid errors in such circumstances **we introduce digital codes to define professions and other qualities**.

The pseudo-quantitative variable may be generated on the basis of the qualitative variable. Let analyze the problem of smoking cigarettes. We can interpret it as qualitative – YES – smoking, NO – no smoking. The rough estimation of the intensity of smoking can be as follows: non-smoking (code 0), occasionally (code 1), permanent low level (code 2), constant smoker (code 3), hard smoker (code 4). As it can be seen the cove value is proportional to the estimated intensity of smoking. This kind of definition of the variable is called **ordinary variable**.

> Anticipating the matter of the later parts of this handbook we suggest that we use the digital codes and ascribe their values in an appropriate way. The values of the codes should be proportional to the variable under consideration. **It is recommended that the features unfavourable for the patient are ascribed to the higher numerical values, and the neutral or favourable features to the lower**. Let e.g. smoking be expressed with number 1, and non-smoking determined by number 0.

> Let us assume that we encode the patient's profession. This feature seems to be neutral. It is proven, though, that from the point of view of the specific illness, there are professions more or less likely to induce the ailment. The numerical value of the code that determines the profession can be assumed proportionally to the given risk factor. The profession that does not include a direct contact with toxic substances (e.g. asbestos) will be encoded with 0 number, while the profession that induces a contact with asbestos will be encoded as 1. The detrimental factors in the profession formulation can obviously be differentiated and depend on the analysed medical problem.

> The exception variable is the gender coding system. The 0–1 (M–F) codes may be applied or just traditionally F and M are the letters to express the patients sex.

If we have already constructed a complete information record, it is time to collect the data. As it has already been told, the information record constitutes a common matrix for each respective patient. The same questions are asked to all the people in identical sequence. The answers (such as the result of body fluids component measurement or an encoded answer concerning the qualitative feature) will be inserted in the suitable and ordered places.

Given below, there is a full record of information and the characteristics of its particular elements.

# A QUESTIONNAIRE

A sample information record with the instruction of filling in the appropriate fields (fragment).

| No | VARIABLE | NOTATION | ANSWERS | | | | | | | |
|---|---|---|---|---|---|---|---|---|---|---|
| 1 | Identification (the case history number) | | P/IIKCh178-32 | | | | | | | |
| 2 | Personal ID number | | 1 | 7 | 2 | 3 | 4 | 8 | 1 | 2 |
| 3 | Family name | | K | O | W | A | L | | | |
| 4 | Name | | A | N | N | | | | | |
| 5 | Address | | | | | | | | | |
| 6 | Insurance Company | | MAŁOPOLSKA | | | | | | | |
| 7 | Gender | M, F | F | | | | | | | |
| 8 | Profession | Insert the right code: 1-miner; 2-cook; 3-sportsman; 4-other; 5-not applicable | 3 | | | | | | | |
| 9 | **Age** | **Number of years** | **33** | | | | | | | |
| 10 | Drink limitation | Y, N | N | | | | | | | |
| 11 | Diet | Insert the right text: Meat; Dairy; Vegetarian | Dairy | | | | | | | |
| 12 | Family record – relatives with the renal ailment | Y, N | Y | | | | | | | |
| 13 | Anatomical defect – patient | Y, N | N | | | | | | | |
| 14 | Anatomical defect specification – patient | Insert the right digital value: 1. Pyelocalyceal narrowing 2. Pyelocalyceal duplication 3. Spongeous kidney 4. Not found | 4 | | | | | | | |
| 15 | Accompanying illnesses | Y, N | N | | | | | | | |
| 16 | Other illnesses: | Insert the right digital code 1. diabetes 2. hypertension 3. ostcoporosis 4. obesity 5. cardiological 6. primary parathyroid gland hyperfunction 7. prostate hypertrophy 8. canccr 9. no illness | 9 | | | | | | | |
| 17 | Diabetes | Y, N | N | | | | | | | |
| 18 | Hypertension | Y, N | N | | | | | | | |
| 19 | Osteoporosis | Y, N | N | | | | | | | |
| 20 | Primary parathyroid gland hyperfunction | Y, N | N | | | | | | | |
| 21 | Cardiovascular diseases | Y, N | N | | | | | | | |

| 22 | Prostate hypertrophy | Y, N | N |
|---|---|---|---|
| 23 | Cancer | Y, N | N |
| 24 | Mobility impairment | Y, N | N |
| 25 | The stone localization | Write the appropriate: Kidney; Ureter; Bladder | Kidney |
| 26 | Localization | 1– multiple site; 2 – single site | 2 |
| 27 | **Urine pH** | **value** | **6.8** |
| 28 | Haematuria | Y, N | Y |
| 29 | The kind of blood cell | 1. lixiviated 2. not lixiviated | 2 |
| 30 | Bacteriuria | Y, N | N |
| 31 | The kind of bacteria | Insert the strain | |
| 32 | The stone composition | Write: Uric acid; Phosphates; Oxalates; Cystine; Xantine | Phosphates |
| 33 | **Temperature** | **Celsius grades** | **36.8** |
| 34 | **$Ca^{++}$ conc. in urine** | **mg%** | **5.1** |
| 35 | **$Mg^{++}$ conc. in urine** | **mg%** | **2.2** |
| 36 | **Urine specific density** | **$g/cm^3$** | **1.021** |
| 37 | **Erythrocytes** | **number/mm$^2$** | **50** |
| 38 | Removal operation type | Surgery – S, lithotripsy – L | L |
| 39 | The first operation | Date dd/mm/yyyy | 03/04/1991 |
| 40 | The second operation | Date dd/mm/yyyy | 16/12/2007 |
| 41 | The censored [4] | Yes – 1; No – 0 | 0 |

*Nota Bene:*
*In the right column, write the right answers according to the pattern given in the column captioned NOTATION. Please fill in the name, surname, and personal ID inserting one letter in one box.*
*Thank you*

**Tab. 1.** The example (fragment) of the form concerning the patients with urolithiasis.[5]

When setting up the database the standard tools can be used (e.g. the Microsoft Office packet) such as the Excel spreadsheet. The entries that determine the positions in the information record are inserted in the first row then. Each column in that kind of arrangement is a set of answers to the given question. The respective rows of the table represent the next patient's set of answers. A fragment of the sample table is shown in Fig. 1.1.

---

[4] The explanation of the notion "censored" will be given in Step 10.
[5] The initial positions that apply to the name, surname, address, and personal ID are used for the patient identification. These data are important for the physician as there is a necessity to keep contact with the patient and for the financial reasons (the questions of the patient's insurance). Those data are not included in the statistical analysis (although they would be important in case the analysis is health service funding oriented).

| H | I | J | K | L | M | N | O |
|---|---|---|---|---|---|---|---|
| AGE | PROFESS. | LOCALIZ. | COMP. | pH | BLOOD IN URINE | BACTERIA IN URINE | TEMP. |
| 47 | 44 | KIDNEY | PHOSPH | 7.3 | N | N | 36.6 |
| 21 | 44 | KIDNEY | OXALATE | 5.2 | N | N | 36.6 |
| 84 | 1 | KIDNEY | OXALATE | 6.9 | Y | Y | 38.3 |
| 46 | 5 | URETER | PHOSPH | 6.5 | N | N | 36.3 |
| 16 | 4 | URETER | PHOSPH | 6.7 | Y | Y | 37 |
| 43 | 5 | KIDNEY | OXALATE | 5.6 | Y | N | 36.4 |
| 39 | 4 | KIDNEY | PHOSPH | 6.1 | Y | Y | 37 |
| 43 | 4 | URETER | PHOSPH | 6.5 | Y | Y | 37 |
| 58 | 4 | KIDNEY | OXALATE | 6.4 | Y | Y | 36.8 |
| 71 | 4 | URETER | CYS | 5.7 | N | Y | 37.2 |
| 90 | 1 | KIDNEY | URICAC | 7.6 | Y | Y | 38.3 |
| 25 | 1 | URETER | PHOSPH | 5.7 | N | Y | 38.6 |
| 53 | 5 | KIDNEY | OXALATE | 5.1 | Y | N | 36.4 |
| 41 | 2 | KIDNEY | OXALATE | 6.5 | Y | Y | 37.8 |
| 65 | 4 | KIDNEY | OXALATE | 6 | Y | Y | 37.2 |
| 49 | 3 | KIDNEY | URICAC | 6.1 | N | Y | 37.4 |
| 27 | 4 | KIDNEY | OXALATE | 6 | Y | N | 36.6 |
| 49 | 3 | KIDNEY | OXALATE | 7.1 | Y | Y | 37.4 |
| 55 | 3 | URETER | PHOSPH | 6 | Y | Y | 37.4 |
| 68 | 4 | KIDNEY | OXALATE | 7.1 | Y | N | 36.8 |
| 51 | 4 | URETER | KSAN | 5.7 | Y | Y | 37 |
| 28 | 1 | BLADDER | PHOSPH | 5.4 | Y | Y | 38.2 |

**Fig. 1.1.** A data base fragment in Excel representation[6]

Sometimes we have at our disposal an accessory data entering programme, which is called the **interface**. The programmer who designs such a tool (a specialized one for a given problem) introduces limitations for the particular entries, disabling entering the wrong symbol (e.g. in case of mistaking the measuring units for the specific feature). A sample model of such an interface is shown in Fig. 1.2.

The accessory programme can be ordered with an information technology specialist, having arranged precisely the conditioning for the specific database (e.g. mutually exclusive settings, measuring units, obligatory information selection, etc.).

---

[6] The database fragment in the Excel representation deserves a commentary. The age was given in the numerical way, expressing how old the patient is. The profession was recorded according to the digital codes given in the questionnaire. The stone localization note was expressed verbally (a sequence of signs can also be understood as the text codes). The stone composition was expressed in a similar way. The urine acidity was given in pH scale. Please note the decimal mark that is expressed with the dot (it depends on the regional settings). The haematuria presence was noted with the sequence of symbols that were recognized by the programme as the text signs (arrangement to the left side of the column). The bacteriuria was also expressed with YES and NO entries (recognized as text by the packet). The temperature given in Celsius grades was recognized by the packet as the digital value (adjustment to the right side of the column). This differentiation is absent from the I – M columns, where the centering was obtained with the adequate cell formatting option.

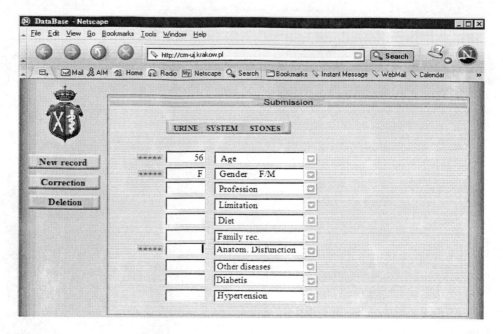

**Fig. 1.2.** A picture of a sample dialogue window (fragment) of the data recording programme with the data correction installed (if a value is inserted in a given window that exceeds the acceptable range for the given measured value, we shall hear a signal and the value will not be entered to the database, most frequently it happens when the measurement units are confused). The scroll option, if activated shows us the recording system for the given feature after each question. The prompt can be given in the dialogue window itself (as it is the case for gender). The red asterisks on the left side of the question show those that are obligatory. If the window with asterisks is left blank, entering the further information is stopped. The present position of the cursor in the picture is in the anatomical disfunction query window. In the left part of the window there is an action choice (at present, the new record introduction)

The programme (interface) for data entering can be designed in the communication system, e.g. through the Internet network, which can be applied in remote way using the appropriate keys (in order to restrict the unauthorized access because of the confidential character of the medical data) that guarantee that the data are classified. It is extremely convenient, not only for the database multiple accessibility (as the data can come in from different hospitals) but also within one hospital, where it enables entering the data from various hospital departments (analytical laboratory, outpatient clinic, treatment room, etc.). A specially designed interface tool is very convenient and nowadays it is recommended that such software is designed for the medical data analysing purposes. **(If the inserted value exceeds the acceptable limits, we get informed by a signal that a correction is necessary).**

# Descriptive analysis

Data storing that was briefly presented in the previous chapter, is, right after the medical problem definition, the most important stage of the statistical analysis.[7] If the data has been collected in the correct way, definitely the most difficult part of the working task has been already done. The statistical analysis needs only the correct clicking and choosing the right options accessible in the statistical packet, which in case of this handbook is the SAS programme.

- **What is our group's characteristics?**
- **We begin the descriptive analysis.**

Perhaps everybody, after a hard work consisting in the data collecting, would ask questions concerning the characteristics of the group of people suffering from the illness.

> E.g.: What is the prevailing age of those who suffer the first symptoms? Is this the young people's illness? Of the middle-aged? And, perhaps only of the old ones? Or, perhaps the patients' age is so much variegated that it is difficult to ascribe that disease entity to a specific age group? Is the incidence rate comparable for both genders? What is the most frequently marked chemical composition of the deposit? How often is the fit accompanied by the temperature rise? Urine obstruction? In how many patients other illnesses, apart from urolithiasis have been diagnosed? And many other questions.

The tool that helps us to obtain the answer to these questions is the ***statistical descriptive analysis***. Before beginning the analysis, it is important to realize the kind of data available in the specific case. Other techniques are used for the analysis of the ***measurable data*** (quantitative), and other to the ***qualitative data*** (not measurable).

---

**The measurable qualities** are characterized by determining ***the central tendency measures*** and ***the dispersion measures***.

---

In case of the **qualitative features** we determine only the ***number of people*** who meet a given condition (e.g. the number of people in whom the bacteria presence in urine has been detected).

---

[7] The available software for the physicians nowadays is differentiated (medical discipline, the Professional position etc) so an independent data preparation is not required. We make use of those data that have been stored by our specialist programme that we made use of throughout our medical practice. The problem can be only limiting the standard way stored data to the form suitable for the given medical subject.

*The measurable feature* (as it is easy to guess) is a feature that is expressed when a certain value, e.g. the patient's age, the stone size, urine pH, urine specific gravity, blood pressure, the number of blood corpuscles in the microscope vision field, etc. is measured. Among the measurable features, we differentiate the *continuous* and *discrete* measurable features. A *continuous measurable feature* is, e.g. age, and *discrete measurable feature is*, e.g. the number of blood corpuscles in the vision field of a microscope image. And how to differentiate between those two features?

> According to the definition, the *continuous measurable feature* is the one that can assume any value from the whole logical range (for the given feature). In other words, there is no such value from that range that is excluded as the given feature measure. There is no logical reason to exclude as impossible e.g. any human body temperature value from 35 do 44 Celsius grade bracket.
>
> In case of the blood corpuscles in the vision field (which can either be completely absent or unlimitedly abundant), there are such values that cannot be that feature measure. Such a value is e.g. 7.8, as the blood cell number can only be integral. So, there are values that are excluded as the measure of the *discrete measurable feature*.

> **Therefore the temperature is the continuous measurable feature, while the red cell number in the vision field is the abrupt measurable feature.**

It should be noted that the thing considered is the character – or nature – of the discussed feature. **It turns out, though, that defining this feature as continuous is only a theoretical specification of its nature. In experimental conditions each feature is practically treated as the discrete feature, though.** The values, which for any sensible range will not appear as the measurement results are those that are beyond the measuring instrument precision. If we ask about the patient's age, we agree to a certain kind of accuracy, e.g. the year. Therefore the number 54.38 (fifty-four and thirty-eight hundredths of a year) will not appear in the database. So the number will not appear in the database, and the patient's age will assume the discrete feature character because of the limited measurement accuracy possibilities. **It does not mean, though, that the age is not a naturally continuous feature.**

A non-measurable (qualitative) feature is e.g. the colour of the eyes, the urine colour, the bacteria presence in urine (YES, NO), the strain of bacteria that appear in urine, the professional activity, etc. in such cases we can only ask how many people represented the given feature. **The qualitative feature can be thus characterized only by giving the number of people that represent it.** The analysis of that feature is extended of course, e.g. to relative forms (in relation to the number of all the analysed cases), as relative sizes (between the particular subgroups), etc. All those estimates are based on the number of cases, though.

**It is possible to change the measurable feature status to the relative feature status.** Here, the example can be the attitude towards the substance concentration in the body fluids. E.g. the calcium salts concentration in urine can be precisely measured in the concentration units, and then it is treated as a measurable feature. However, if the level of calcium compounds in urine is higher than the accepted norm (above 5 mm mol/l), it signifies the hypercalciuria case in the patient. The information of the acceptable level exceeding can be expressed either as a case of hypercalciuria (YES), which signifies exceeding a certain level, or the illness absence (NO), which signifies the concentration lower than the established limit. **We have quitted the measurable character of the feature that is the substance concentration and assumed the qualitative classification. It does not mean, though, that the nature of such a feature as the concentration has been changed. We have only changed the form in which we refer to that feature.** That division is good in the cases when the withdrawal from the exact measurement of the given measurable feature does not influence the final result and we do not need the exact knowledge of the afore-said feature.[8]

On summarizing the feature characteristics, their kind should be differentiated:
1. measurable (quantitative) – the measuring units (e.g.: kg, cm, etc.)
    a. continuous,
    b. discrete,
2. non-measurable (qualitative), sometimes defined as discrete.
    a. ordinal,
    b. non-ordinal

Coming back to our information record, the measurable properties in the questionnaire record (information record) were marked as boldface.[9]

- **We analyse the measurable variables**

If a given feature is being measured, we probably would like to learn the value that is most representative for the measurement results. We would also like to learn how much the results of a certain value measurement are dispersed.

> **The descriptive analysis of the measurable features** satisfies our curiosity in two ways: from the point of view of the values that contain all the values that are in the given data base defined by means of the so-called *central tendency measures*, and the value of dispersion expressed with *dispersion measures*.

While discussing the ways of calculating the local tendency measure values (arithmetic mean) and dispersion, two formulae will be introduced. One of them will specify the theoretical value of the parameter (the so-called **parameter for population**), while the next one will present the way of calculating the given parameter with respect to the specific community (the so-called **parameter for the sample**).

---

[8] Sometimes the decision of the qualitative record of the measurable variable can result from the necessity of reducing the analysis costs in case of very expensive quantitative measurements.

[9] The information record contains all the position included in the analysis. A questionnaire is a form of information recording with respect to the remarks and the instructions needed for its correct filling in. The paper questionnaire forms are being replaced by the computer recording.

The *local tendency measures* are defined by the following parameters:
1. The *arithmetic mean* ($\mu$) and ($\overline{x}$) – the sum of all the elements divided by the number of the elements in the set:

$$\mu = \frac{\sum\limits_{i=1}^{N} x_i}{N} \qquad \text{(eq. 1.1.)}$$

$$\overline{x} = \frac{\sum\limits_{i=1}^{n} x_i}{n}, \qquad \text{(eq. 1.2.)}$$

where $N$ **expresses a(n) (unknown) number of elements in the population, n – the number of elements in the sample,** $x_i$ signifies the respective values of the elements in a sample.

As it has already been mentioned, the formula (1.1.) expresses the definition of the notion rather than the way of calculating it, that is given with the 1.2. equation. **The given differentiation of meaning** $N$ (the population number) **and** *n* (the known sample number) **will be obligatory in the whole handbook.**
2. *Median* (Me) – in order to find the median value, all the values expressing the given feature measure should be ordered (in ascending or descending order). The middle (central) value *in the ordered series* **is precisely the median**. If the series consists of the even number of values, the median is the arithmetic mean of the two middle values in the series.
3. *Modal or mode* (Mo) – **value, which has appeared the most often in the analysed series of values that constitute the measurement result of a given feature in the tested group**. If two, three or even more values in the series appear with the same highest frequency, we call the series two-, three-, or four-modal.

**NOTA BENE**
There is a frequent mistake made by students, especially while looking for the median! **One must not remove the results with the same values!** In the ordered series, each patient must be present and must not be omitted for the sole reason, that the result of measuring a certain feature is the same as in another patient.
The second very frequent, unacceptable error is calculating arithmetic mean for the encoded values. Although we try to encode the qualitative features in a certain determined order (e.g.: different occupations are symbolized with the codes of the values growing along with the threatening danger level growth, e.g. from the toxic substances), still by no means we can treat those codes as the measure of anything. If we encode e.g. the feminine gender as –1, and the masculine as –2, the calculated arithmetic mean e.g. 1.58 signifies nothing.

The definition of *central tendency measurement* is connected with localizing on the number axis the values that constitute the measurement results, (e.g. the Papuan pygmies' stature will be found on the number axis in the section representing numbers close to 100 cm; while the basketball players' stature will be found close to the values of 200 cm).

The points that represent the given set of values expressing the measurement result and at the same time specifying the situation on the number axis are: the *arithmetic mean, median*, and the *modal (mode)*. The numerical values of the enumerated parameters and especially the relation between them characterize the set of values in an approximate way. The special case is such a situation, when all those values ($\bar{x}$, Me, Mo) are equal. We are going to return to this problem in the further part of the book.

Apart from the situation measures (and so the values specifying the situation on the number axis), it is interesting to learn the dispersion value of the measured feature. We define the characteristics of the given feature as *the dispersion (spread) measures*. Those measures are:

1. The *interval* (R) – the difference between the highest and the lowest value in the data series that constitute the given feature measurement result:

$$R = x_{max} - x_{min} \qquad \text{(eq. 1.3.)}$$

2. The *variance* ($\sigma^2$, $s^2$) – specifies an average of the total squared dispersion between each observation and arithmetic mean:

$$\sigma^2 = \frac{\sum_{i=1}^{N}(x_i - \mu)^2}{N} \qquad \text{(eq. 1.4.)}$$

$$s^2 = \frac{\sum_{i=1}^{n}(x_i - \bar{x})^2}{n-1} \qquad \text{(eq. 1.5.)}$$

3. The *standard deviation* ($\sigma$, $s$) is the square root from the variance:

$$\sigma = \sqrt{\sigma^2} = \sqrt{\frac{\sum_{i=1}^{N}(x_i - \mu)^2}{N}} \qquad \text{(eq. 1.6.)}$$

$$s = \sqrt{s^2} = \sqrt{\frac{\sum_{i=1}^{n}(x_i - \bar{x})^2}{n-1}} \qquad \text{(eq. 1.7.)}$$

**The interval** is the intuitively evident value and everybody would suggest such a measure without any particular difficulties.

**Variance** is the value that expresses the medium square of the difference between the mean values and the measurement results. There are certain problems with that value. They consist in the fact that that the dimension of this parameter is the square of the measured unit, so if we want to learn the value of the patients' age dispersion, we get the number of the years' square (WE GET THE RESULT IN THE YEARS TO THE SECOND POWER). Such a value is impossible to interpret. Calculating the values of the standard deviation is the problem's solution (SOLVES THE PROBLEM). Having calculated the square root of the variance we obtain the value, whose dimension agrees with the dimension of the measured value.

The formulas for variance (1.4., 1.5.) and standard deviation (1.6., 1.7.) (according to the notation given earlier) present the theoretical definitions for the population (1.4. and 1.6.) and the way of calculating the values for those parameters for the specific sample of the known size (1.5., 1.7.).

> Moderately anticipating the facts, variance is a very important parameter in statistical analysis and will be very frequently referred to in the further part of the handbook. Nevertheless, whenever the scattering of a given value is interpreted, the standard deviation value is interpreted.
>
> It is also necessary to explain the denominator character in the variance formula for the sample. The value $n-1$ signifies the number of degrees freedom for the sample. As it has already been said, one parameter – mean value – has been already defined, the number of freedom degrees for this sample had been diminished by one before.[10]

- **The confidence interval**

We have already said that only a sample is accessible for the analysis and not the whole population. If we know the calculated arithmetic mean or another measure of the central tendency or dispersion, then it represents only the drawn sample. We can intuitively foresee that drawing a slightly different group (sample) of patients can cause the appearance of the different values of those parameters. What confidence interval can we have with respect to the assigned parameters of our sample? The question is answered by a certain calculation type, which enables us to estimate not only the value of a specific parameter, but also the value of the interval (range) in which there is a considerable probability of the appearance of the parameter value analysed by e.g. arithmetic mean irrespectively of the next sample component drawing. That kind of interval is called the *confidence interval*.

The procedure of calculating the values for the confidence interval deserves knowledge of certain notions which are going to be presented in the further part of the handbook. For the time being it is enough to assimilate the notion and understand its meaning.

---

[10] There is another mathematical justification of the expression $n-1$. It can be found in each statistics handbook. Yet it needs the professional knowledge of those matters that are beyond the scope of this handbook.

The confidence interval (defined by its upper and lower limit) on the level of e.g. 95% for the values such as the standard deviation, states the range in which, with the probability 95% there is the value standard deviation for the given population Without knowing the values' standard deviation for the population, we are satisfied with the values confidence interval in which the value of the standard deviation (or of another parameter) is found with a certain probability (e.g. 95%).

Another measure that specifies for us the range of the measured values is specifying the so-called quartile.

The first quartile is the value of the measured value that cuts off lowest 25% of data (which is to say the least quarter – the least quartile).

Median – which also is called the second quartile (or $50^{th}$ percentile – see below) specifies the measured value that cuts off half of lowest values from the top ones.

The third quartile (or $75^{th}$ percentile) cuts off those values, that constitute the ¾ of all the measurements in the ordered set, cutting only ¼ of the highest results.

The quartile divides the whole sample into 4 parts. If we are interested in the other ranges, we turn to calculating the so-called **percentiles** – a percentile is the value of a variable below which a certain percent of observations fall.

That way the $60^{th}$ percentile is the value that cuts off lowest 60% of all the results (in the ordered series).

The ways of calculating all the characteristics (Fig. 1.3.) described here with the SAS packet are given in the workbook part. Here the discussed parameters have been grouped together to describe the data concerning the analysed patients only.

|  | MEAN | Me | Mo | N | MIN | MAX | RANGE | VARIANCE | ST. DEV. |
|---|---|---|---|---|---|---|---|---|---|
| AGE | 44.47 | 46 | 36 | 256 | 4 | 94 | 90 | 326.37 | 18.07 |
| TEMP | 36.97 | 37 | 36.8 | 256 | 36 | 39.2 | 3.2 | 0.42 | 0.65 |
| pH | 7.9 | 6.3 | 6.1 | 256 | 5.1 | 7.9 | 2.8 | 0.53 | 0.73 |
| PHOSPHATE | 44.6 | 39 | 45 | 248 | 16 | 48 | 32 | 26.01 | 5.1 |
| $Mg^{2+}$ | 1.8 | 1.8 | 1.9 | 231 | 1.5 | 7.5 | 6 | 0.64 | 0.8 |
| URICATE | 4.1 | 3.81 | 4.2 | 250 | 2.38 | 4.46 | 2.08 | 1.21 | 1.1 |
| OXALATE | 0.51 | 0.5 | 0.5 | 250 | 0.4 | 0.6 | 0.2 | 0.01 | 0.1 |
| $Ca^{2+}$ | 6.1 | 4.6 | 4.8 | 213 | 0.25 | 7.5 | 7.25 | 1.44 | 1.2 |
| DENSITY | 1.023 | 1.02 | 1.02 | 228 | 1 | 1.03 | 0.025 | 0.00014 | 0.012 |

**Fig. 1.3.** A sample set of the situation measures and the dispersion measures for the values present in our database

Analysing the given table and the following the nephrolithiasis patients' group description tells us that this is an illness that occurs in the group of the middle-aged people – 44.5 years old, although the large interval and the standard deviation suggest, that in the group of patients there are also both very young people and those whose age is very advanced. The body temperature mean value suggests that, the illness is not accompanied by very high temperatures (the value standard deviation is also low). In contrary to the age situation measures, the situation measures, of the body temperature are very close to each other. The arithmetic mean, median and modal (e.g. for the temperature) equality will be interpreted in the further part of the book.

### The qualitative variables:

The qualitative features, as it has already been told, are characterized only by giving the number of cases. They can be given in the absolute numbers they can also be given in the relative numbers (frequencies) (Fig. 1.4. and Fig. 1.5.).

|  | Y | N |
|---|---|---|
| BACTERIA IN URINE | 165 | 91 |
| BLOOD IN URINE | 187 | 69 |
| PNP | 7 | 249 |
| IMMOBIL. | 28 | 228 |
| DRINK LIMITATION | 70 | 186 |
| CANCER | 29 | 227 |
|  | F | M |
| GENDER | 94 | 162 |

**Fig. 1.4.** An example of the qualitative data description by means of giving the number of people who satisfy the given condition (Y – yes), and those who do not satisfy it (N – no)

| | PHOSPHATE | OXALATE | URIC ACID | CYS | KSANT | | |
|---|---|---|---|---|---|---|---|
| COMPOUND | 80 | 88 | 80 | 6 | 2 | | |
| | DIABETES | HIPERTENS. | OSTEOP. | OBESITY | HEART | CANCER | NO |
| OTHER DISEASE | 38 | 39 | 25 | 51 | 21 | 31 | 25 |
| | PYELOC. OBSTR. | PYELOC. DUPLIC. | SPONGEOUS | NO | | | |
| ANATOM. DIS. | 92 | 52 | 7 | 105 | | | |
| | MINER | COOK | SPORT | OTHER | | | |
| PROFESSION | 44 | 21 | 12 | 143 | | | |
| | KIDNEY | URETER | BLADDER | | | | |
| LOCALIZATION | 167 | 70 | 19 | | | | |
| | DAIRY | MEAT | WEGET | | | | |
| DIET | 46 | 66 | 144 | | | | |

**Fig. 1.5.** Setting the number of people in the groups of patients with respect to the different versions of qualifying the patient

The proportion of women to men among the patients suggests that urolithiasis hits mainly men. Urolithiasis appears more frequently in the people whose family members also suffered from it. A limited access to drinks is reported by a lower number of patients. It is also interesting to analyse the frequency of other illness occurrence in the patients suffering from urolithiasis.

The characteristics of the patients' diet indicates that the most numerous group are vegetarians.

The most numerous group among the patients, in whom other illness cases were found, are those with obesity.

Among the most frequently observed urinary system anatomical changes the obstructive pyelocalyceal uropathy was found.

The table analysis shows also that urolithiasis is frequently accompanied by the urinary tract inflammation. The majority of patients has deposits in various places of the urinary tract. Urolithiasis fits are frequently accompanied by haematuria.

The analysis of the crystalline deposit composition shows that the particular salts occur with the comparable frequency. The occurrence of the cystine and xanthine stones is the least frequently observed.

The description of the patients group was based upon the measures of central tendency and dispersion and the measurable features calculation.

The patient group characteristics with respect to the qualitative features was made by analysing the numbers of patients that represented the particular conditions (frequency).

# Exercises

When you will have studied the workbook part, perform the following tasks:

1. Characterize the information record specified for the data concerning traffic injuries (the CD attached to the handbook), enumerating the qualitative and quantitative features with the differentiation between the constant and the abrupt ones.
2. Ask a question concerning the traffic accident victims that you would like to be answered by making a statistical analysis of the data on the CD.
3. Characterize the population that is represented by the database on the CD.
4. Construct the ordered series with respect to the feature that is important from the point of view of the selected issue describing the problem of traffic accidents.
5. Determine the measures of central tendency and dispersion of those measurable features, whose analysis is important from the point of view of the question asked in 2.
6. Specify the number of people who belong to the groups whose analysis is important for the problem chosen in 2. Present the frequencies of patients in respect to qualitative variables.

# STEP 1 – exercise

# Preliminary data analysis

This part shows how to use particular programs to perform the analysis of data collected describing the set of patients who are under our consideration. Two tools will be presented: Excel program (commonly available as the part of Microsoft Office) and professional statistical program called SAS.

The aim to present the calculations performed using Excel is to show that all operations are very easy and any person without special preparation is able to do it. The self-performance is also to show that there are neither secrets nor black magic in mathematical/statistical calculations. The self-performance is also to help the understanding of all operations.

The use of professional program (which is SAS in this manual) is aimed to present the high level tool used by specialists. The medical student experiences the calculations done by him/her self to understand the methodology applied in statistical analysis to know what to expect as the results of statistical procedures and how to interpret the decisions and conclusion based on the estimation procedures.

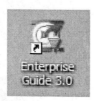

**Fig. 1.1.** By clicking on the SAS icon on your computer's desktop, you get into the SAS program

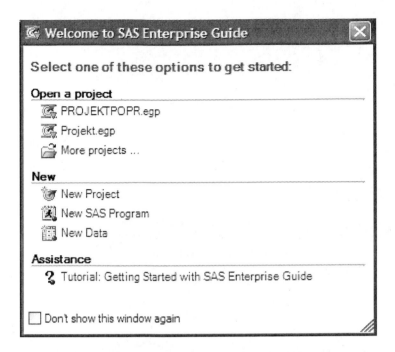

**Fig. 1.2.** After starting the program, SAS opens a window to select a new session or continue previous sessions. In our example we select New Project

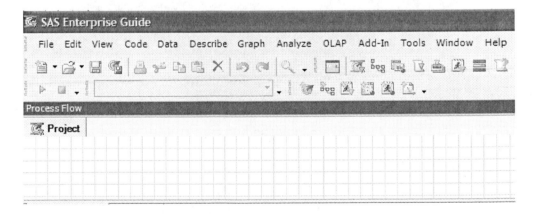

**Fig. 1.3.** Toolbars in the SAS dialog box are similar to those in typical MS Windows applications. Certain icons, especially those related to editing are identical. New items on the toolbar are related to data analysis. Below the toolbar there is a communication box in which the system informs us about the manipulation of data

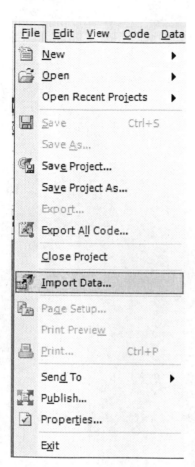

**Fig. 1.4.** Each session begins with loading a dataset, which – as in our example – has been saved as an Excel file. We select an Import Data option. If the dataset is saved using the SAS package, we select an Open option

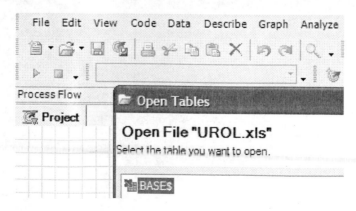

**Fig. 1.5.** The dataset is called UROL and the communication box contains a message saying which file is used. The Import Data window helps us to specify the conditions of data loading

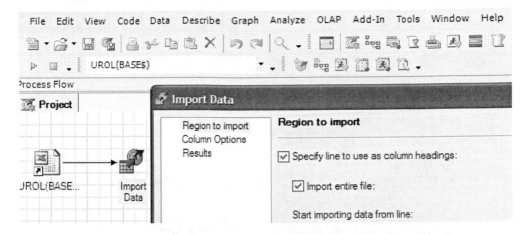

**Fig. 1.6.** After loading the data, columns of the database are displayed in the lower part of the screen. Data loading starts with the appearance of the SASUSER icon. The headline contains the names of variables (characteristics) and symbols that differentiate the status of the variable – the red pyramid identifies a qualitative characteristic and the blue ball a measurable characteristic. An ID (identifier), which is a numerical symbol, has been qualified as a measurable characteristic, but it is of no importance in this case. First and last names, addresses and personal identification numbers (PESEL) have been skipped because they will not be used in our analysis

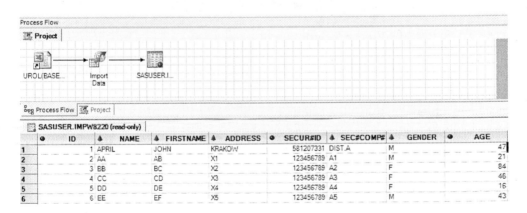

**Fig. 1.7.** The lower scrollbar (the same as in Excel) scrolls the window that displays the data. Numerical codes related to diet type and professions have been incorrectly identified as measurable characteristics. By pressing the right mouse button you access Edit options

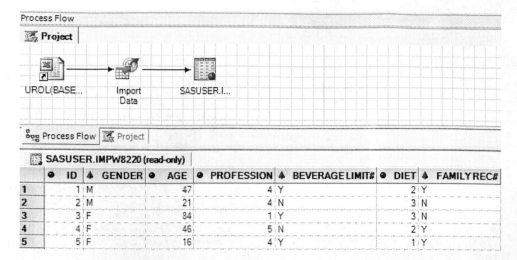

Process Flow

Project

UROL(BASE...      Import        SASUSER.I...
                  Data

Process Flow   Project

SASUSER.IMPW8220 (read-only)

| | ID | GENDER | AGE | PROFESSION | BEVERAGE LIMIT# | DIET | FAMILY REC# |
|---|---|---|---|---|---|---|---|
| 1 | 1 | M | 47 | 4 | Y | 2 | Y |
| 2 | 2 | M | 21 | 4 | N | 3 | N |
| 3 | 3 | F | 84 | 1 | Y | 3 | N |
| 4 | 4 | F | 46 | 5 | N | 2 | Y |
| 5 | 5 | F | 16 | 4 | Y | 1 | Y |

**Fig. 1.8.** Same database worksheet as is appears after removal of personal data. The personal data are necessary for the doctor to contact patients. They are useless for statistical analysis. The database without personal data shall be delivered to the specialists in statistics to make the calculation anonymous

# STEP 2

# We analyse the distribution of the measurable variable

Σ

Summary
Statistics

**What type of distribution is presented by the clinical measurable variables?**
**Why is finding the distribution type of the measurable feature essential?**
**Is the female patients' age distribution comparable to the male patients' age distribution?**

In the previous chapter, we learned the values that characterize the measurable feature from the point of view of the situation measures and the distribution, although it is not the complete characteristics of the measurable feature yet. It is not known how many people represent very high values and how many people represent very low ones; e.g. if there is a majority of young people in the group, or, if there is any age group that is particularly numerous within the whole group of patients. Those questions are answered by our distribution type analysis. The question concerning the distribution type can be substituted for the question concerning the distribution of the particular results distribution in the range between the highest and the lowest value in the set of measurements.

So, another step of the analysis is estimating the *measured variable distribution*. Expressing it exactly – the distribution specifies in a general way the change of frequency of a given measured value occurrence with respect to its value.

To provide an example of the distribution type analysis we shall make, exact calculations for the male and female patients age in our data base.

If the distribution of the given measurable feature is known, we can also learn e.g. the probability degree of meeting a 17-year old person or the probability degree of meeting a person of 70 up to 75, which is to say, a person of the given age (or another measurable feature), or a person that belongs to the determined age group. Such information is particularly important for e.g. the hospital head, who, having learnt the age distribution from the group description of those patients who are already present in the hospital ward, can estimate the demand for the rehabilitation equipment for the aged people.

The "distribution specification" is a short form of its correct full version, namely: "the probability of meeting a given value (or belonging to the assigned range)".

However, before it is possible to conduct the complete analysis, we shall learn the notions connected with the calculus of probability.

The **definition of probability** of some event $E$ applied for our discussion can be presented with a simple expression:

$$P(E) = \frac{M}{N} \qquad \text{(eq. 2.1.)}$$

$$P(E) = \frac{m}{n}, \qquad \text{(eq. 2.2.)}$$

where $m$ signifies the number of solutions favourable from the point of view of a given analysis (e.g. finding the person without an accompanying illness, which is, e.g. osteoporosis, while $n$ – the total number of outcomes, including the unfavourable ones (in our case it signifies the total number of people in the sample). The symbols $M$ and $N$ signify the numbers adequate with respect to the population.

In order to extend the knowledge of the probability calculus notions, certain essential properties shall be presented.

In our group of patients who suffer from renal colic, are those who work as cooks, there are professional sportsmen, but there are also other professions. We can ask, then, about the probability of drawing from the patients group someone who works as a miner. We know that there are 44 of them in our group ($m = 44$). The whole sample (number of people present in the analysis) is 256, so $n = 256$. The probability of the occurrence of a miner in our sample is equal 44/256. We know that the drink access limitation and strong perspiration are likely to cause nephrolithiasis. So, if we ask about the probability of meeting someone who is a miner or a ship cook, we shall find the answer on the basis of the probabilities of the union of events (with assumption that events are mutually exclusive).

$$P(E_i \text{ or } E_j) = P(F_i \cup F_j) = P(E_i) + P(E_j) \qquad \text{(eq. 2.3.)}$$

$$P(miner \text{ or } cook) = 44/256 + 21/256 = 65/256 = 0.254 \qquad \text{(eq. 2.4.)}$$

The probability of the union can be extended to any components number (with the same assumption as above).

$$P(E_1 \ or \ E_2 \ or \cdots or \ E_n) = P(E_1 \cup E_2 \cup \cdots \cup E_n) = P(E_1) + P(E_2) + \cdots + P(E_n)$$

(eq. 2.5.)

In special case when events $E_1$, $E_2$, ..., $E_n$ are mutually exclusive and the sum total of these events is equal to the probability space this sum of probabilities is equal to 1.

$$P(E_1 \ or \ E_2 \ or \cdots or \ E_n) = P(E_1) + P(E_2) + \cdots + P(E_n) = 1 \qquad \text{(eq. 2.5.a)}$$

If we assume that the cause of nephrolithiasis appearance in the sportsmen is also intensive perspiration that accompanies an intensive physical effort (and loose of water), the question about the probability of meeting in the analysed sample people whose professions are connected with intensive perspiration, the probability of such an event will be calculated in the following way:

$$P(perspiration) = P(cook) + P(miner) + P(sportsman) \qquad \text{(eq. 2.6.)}$$

$$= 21/256 + 44/256 + 12/256 = 77/256 = 0.30 \qquad \text{(eq. 2.7.)}$$

Conducting the above calculations, we made use of the probabilities of an alternative, expressed in a symbolic way with the equation (eq. 2.3.). The principle says that finding a person who meets the condition $E_1$ (professional cook) or condition $E_2$ (miner) is expressed with the sum of the probabilities of finding independently a person who meets the $E_1$ criterion and, independently, the $E_2$ criterion. We have to mind the fact that both the subgroups belong to the same group, according to which ($n$) we calculate the partial probability. In general, this is the so-called probability space. The probability space or a sample space in our case is the set of $n$ elements, which all have the same ($1/n$) probability of being drawn.[11] The event in probability theory is a set of outcomes (any subset of a sample space).

The concept of the so-called **mutually exclusive events** is also connected with the question discussed above. The sum of probabilities mentioned above is applicable only to the mutually exclusive events. In our example it can be expressed with a statement that a given patient represents only one profession.

The sum of the values of the probability to meet the patients whose jobs are, respectively: cook, miner, sportsman or an unemployed (i.e. all those that were enumerated in the questionnaire), equals 1. The probability equal to 1 means the certainty. If we ask about the probability of meeting in our sample a miner or a person that represents another profession, or someone who has no professional training, a sportsman or a cook, it will be proved that whoever we draw, we shall always be successful, irrespectively of a particular person drawn from our sample.

Characterizing the relations between the events, one should mention also the notion of mutually exclusive (or mutually complementary) events. A classic example can be the patient's gender specification (we eliminate the cases of gender specification disor-

---

[11] There is also a principle of multiplying the probability values. It concerns expressing the probability event occurrence that meets two conditions simultaneously. In our example the question could concern the probability of drawing a person who is both a miner and a shop cook. A detailed explanation of numerous complexities connected with this example is beyond the scope of this handbook. We can recommend the Reader other handbook upon this subject.

ders). The sum of probabilities of the event $A$ (drawing a woman among the patients) and the contrary event $\overline{A}$ (the circumflex over the symbol $A$ means "*non-A*", which is to say an event contrary to the event $A$ in our example: not drawing a woman, i.e. drawing a man) equals 1. The events currently discussed are specific also as the complementary events. Another example of the complementary events that apply to our example is: A – drawing a person with the bacteria found in his/her urine and $\overline{A}$ – a person without the bacteria found in his/her urine, which constitutes the complementary arrangement. Such examples could be multiplied, e.g. referring to the questions with YES or NO answers.

In order to explain also the events connected with the boundary cases, we shall remind, that $P = 0$ means certainty that the given event does not take place (e.g. the probability of drawing an alien from the group of the analysed patients is so far equal to 0). In the similar way, the probability of drawing a *homo sapiens* from our group of patients equals 1, as all the patients meet that condition.

Analysing these data, we can specify, that:

The probability of encountering in our group of patients a person, whose family has already been troubled with the nephrolithiasis occurrence, is $P = 139/256 = 0.54$, which can be interpreted as more than a half of the ailments connected with the urinary tract function occur with the patients' family members.

If we ask about the probability of encountering among the patients a person who suffers from osteoporosis, then:

$$P = 25/256 = 0.098 \qquad \text{(eq. 2.8.)}$$

The probability of encountering a person who does not suffer from osteoporosis, equals:

$$P = 231/256 = 0.902 \qquad \text{(eq. 2.9.)}$$

One can check, that the sum of the probability values of the event A (there is osteoporosis) and the contrary event – $\overline{A}$ (there is no osteoporosis, so the events are mutually complementary), is equal to the numerical value one. It signifies, that if we ask about the probability of encountering a person with osteoporosis or a person without osteoporosis, whoever we draw then, the drawing result will always meet the expectations, and eventually the success probability equals 1 (because in this case $m$ equals $n$, and eventually $m/n$ is one).

It is important to specify the probability space, which is to say the number of solutions that are taken into account in the given case. If we ask about the probability of meeting a person with the prostate hypertrophy, then the female patients should be excluded from such calculation. Hence:

$$P = 26/162 = 0.16 \qquad \text{(eq. 2.10.)}$$

Number 162 appears in the denominator, as there is only that number of male patients in our group (the probability space is represented by 162 elements). We excluded from the event space drawing a woman, as a person, whom the illness does not affect (as women do not enter the event space connected with prostate hypertrophy).

**The Gaussian function**

We return to the measurable analysis. As it is easy to guess, we shall more often en-
counter the result close to the arithmetic mean value than the result extremely different
from it.

The probability distribution, in which meeting both high and low values is not considerable and mutually comparable with a high probability of meeting the values close
to the arithmetic mean, is the normal distribution expressed with the Gaussian function.[12]

This function has the following form:

$$G(x) = \frac{1}{\sigma\sqrt{2\pi}} \cdot e^{-\frac{(x-\mu)^2}{2\sigma^2}} , \qquad \text{(eq. 2.11.)}$$

where: $\mu$ – arithmetic mean,
$\sigma$ – standard deviation,
$e, \pi$ – mathematical constants.

The graphic form of this function presentation is shown below:

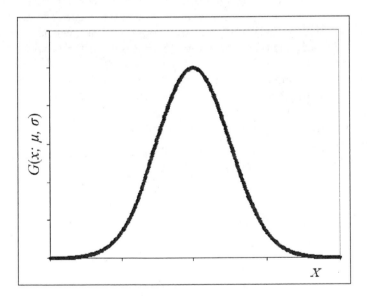

**Fig. 2.1.** An example of the probability distribution created with the 2.11. formula

In its graphic form, the Gauss function assumes a characteristic symmetrical shape of
the bell curve. The maximum of this function is achieved for the value which is marked

---

[12] The principle of summing up the probability values applies only to mutually exclusive
events. If the cook were a miner at the same time, it would be impossible to calculate the simple
sum of probability values. This case is not discussed in this project.

in the formula as $\mu$ and interpreted as the arithmetic mean. With moving away from that value, the probability drops, reaching the values close to zero for the values considerably different from the arithmetic mean (very high and very low).

The Gauss function can be enumerated in the set of the mathematical functions specifying the relation between the independent variable $X$ and the dependent variable $Y$. There are many various functions that can express any instance of such dependence. Some of them have a physical meaning, other are abstract functions. The Gauss function is a specific function, whose interpretation helps to specify the probability $Y$ of appearing the given value $X$. The Gauss function has a theoretical character, the collection of the function arguments can be any from the real numbers set. The function parameters (the arithmetic mean and the standard deviation) can assume any real values (the standard deviation, with respect to its definition – the root square – assumes only the positive values). The Gauss function presents a theoretical probability distribution for a hypothetical population of infinite number of elements in the $X$ set. The parameters of this function are expressed as $\mu$ and $\sigma$, according to the accepted notation.

There are premises, while discussing distribution of the feature value that constitutes the living system functioning element (e.g. the metabolism product concentration in the cell), to expect the distribution following the Gauss function. The metabolite concentrations in the organism fluids result from the processes that underlie a constant control within the so-called homeostasis, according to the negative feedback. The negative feedback consists in the fact that the regulation cycle allows neither too high, nor too low concentrations. The concentrations of products of the processes taking place within the negative feedback frame around the optimal (mean) value are the most probable. Hence, it is extremely important to check if, in case of a given feature analysis, we deal with the distribution keeping the expected distribution according to the Gauss function. If, with respect to a given factor (the body fluid component) we do not notice such distribution, a profound reflection upon the cause of that should be made. In this book, we are going to make returns to the issue of concord or discord of a given feature with the Gaussian distribution many times.

The above notation describing the population (the parameter values are unknown) is also specific as the *theoretical distribution for the population*.

If we apply the above formula to the sample description (the parameter values are known), it assumes the following form (in the notation of the function that specifies the distribution in the sample, the Latin alphabet symbols were used):

$$G(x;\bar{x},s) = \frac{1}{s\sqrt{2\pi}} \cdot e^{-\frac{(x-\bar{x})^2}{2s^2}} \qquad \text{(eq. 2.12.)}$$

This is the notation of the *normal distribution* – of the $\bar{x}, s$ parameters – so the one that describes the distribution features in the sample.

Fig. 2.2. presents the influence of the values standard deviation upon the function shape. The differences between these two distribution types will be analysed in the further part of the handbook.

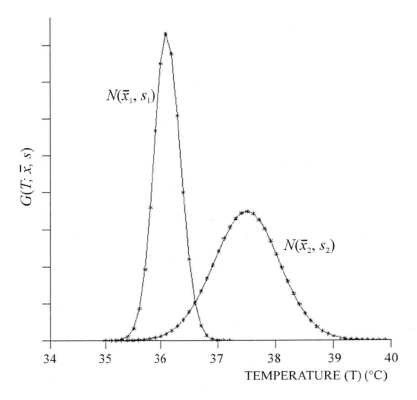

**Fig. 2.2.** Normal distributions for the varied parameters of $\bar{x}$ and $s$

The distribution $N(\bar{x}_1, s_1)$ differs from the distribution $N(\bar{x}_2, s_2)$ both with respect to the mean, which is higher for the sample marked as 2, and the standard deviation value that is higher for the sample marked as 2.

An analysis of the normal distribution function graph (symbolically written down with the letter $N$ and in the parentheses the value of the arithmetical mean and the standard deviation) further explains the mean specification as the central tendency measure (as the localization on the axis depends on that value). The analysis illustrates also the influence of the value $s$ – standard deviation.

The higher the $s$, the lower and wider the bell curve is. Anticipating the further analysis of the Gauss function graphs one can say that the sum of the area under the curve depicts the probability of meeting the values from the min to max and it equals 1. The surface value under the curve is uniform and it is assumed that it equals exactly 1.[13] The variability of the Gauss curve shape is very high nevertheless the surface size under it is standardized.

A role analysis of the $\sigma$ or $s$ parameters has become the basis to determine the so-called three-sigmas rule.

---

[13] Exactly speaking the integrate of the limits $(-\infty, +\infty)$.

The rule will be discussed with the reference to the Gauss function graphs analysis.[14]

The analysis of the normal distribution (as well as the Gauss function) enables presenting a certain characteristics. As it was told earlier, the function maximum value is
achieved for the values $X = \mu$.[15]

The standard deviation is specified as the half width. This signifies, that if we mark
a point that specifies half the maximum value and draw a line parallel to the X-axis,
this line will cross the graph curve in two points, for which the values read on the
X-axis are $\mu + \sigma$ and $\mu - \sigma$,[16] which is to say the axis part between the situation of the
values $\mu$ and the point read as described above marks the standard deviation value.

The normal distribution has many specific features:

1. The graphic interpretation of the function that represents the normal distribution
   enables reading that function's parameters:
   A – the function maximum is reached for the $x$ equal to $\bar{x}$. It signifies, that if
   one reads the value $x$ on the X-axis, for which the maximum has occurred,
   one will thereby read the arithmetic mean;
   B – however, if one divides by two the line connecting the maximum to X-axis,
   and the next one reads all the $x$ values below the points of crossing the line
   parallel to the X-axis with the graph line, the appropriate $x$ values signify
   values $\bar{x} + s$ and $\bar{x} - s$.[17]
2. The area marked in point 1B between $\bar{x} + s$ and $\bar{x} - s$ has a certain property.
   That is a fact, that the probability of meeting values from this range equals 0.68,
   which was graphically presented in Fig. 2.3.a.

---

[14] If $G(x, \bar{x}, s)$ is the probability density function for normal distribution, the half-width $d$ is
the solution of the equation: $\tfrac{1}{2} G(x, \bar{x}, s) = G(x + d, \bar{x}, s)$ which is $d = \pm s\sqrt{2\log 2} = \pm s \cdot 1.17741$.

[15] For $x = \mu \pm \sigma$ function $G$ decreases to the value : $\dfrac{1}{\sqrt{e}} = 0.60653$.

[16] Calculating precisely: $\mu + \sigma\sqrt{2\log 2}$ and $\mu - \sigma\sqrt{2\log 2}$.

[17] Exactly $\bar{x} \pm 1.17741 \cdot s$.

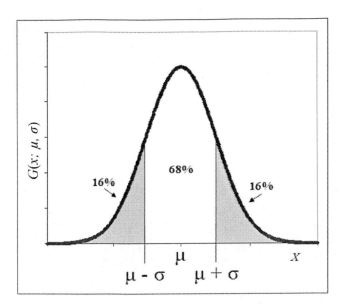

**Fig. 2.3.a.** The three-sigmas rule presented graphically – the range specified with the values $\mu - \sigma$ and $\mu + \sigma$ represents the range of $X$ values, whose probability of meeting equals 68%

3.  If we repeat the procedure shown in 1B point and mark the area limited with the values $\bar{x} - 2s$ and $\bar{x} + 2s$, we shall thus mark the area, for which the value of probability equals 0.95, which is shown in Fig. 2.3.b.

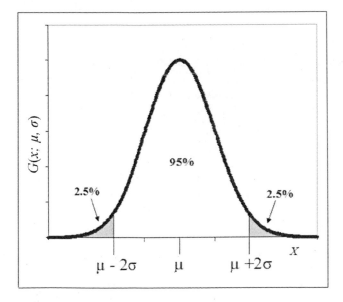

**Fig. 2.3.b.** The three-sigmas rule presented graphically – the range specified with the values $\mu - 2\sigma$ and $\mu + 2\sigma$ represents the range of $X$ values, whose probability of meeting equals 95%

4. If we repeat the procedure again mark the area limited with the values $\bar{x} - 3s$ and $\bar{x} + 3s$, we shall thus mark the area of the probability value 0.997, which was shown in Fig. 2.3.c.

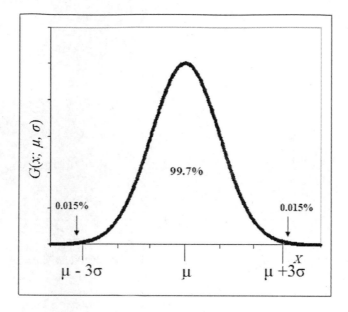

**Fig. 2.3.c.** The three-sigmas rule presented graphically – the range specified with the values $\mu - 3\sigma$ and $\mu + 3\sigma$ represents the range of $X$ values, whose probability of meeting equals 99.7%

The operations presented in Fig. 2.3.a, 2.3.b and 2.3.c are specified together with the so-called three-sigmas rule name. The ranges specified are very frequently used in medical practice to specify the so-called norm ranges. If we say that the optimum diastolic blood pressure is 80 mmHg, but the acceptable normal blood pressure is that of the 70–90 range, that range was defined just upon the basis of the three-sigmas rule. Usually, the range $\bar{x} + s$ and $\bar{x} - s$ are assumed as the range that defines the norm.[18]

The graphic interpretation of the Gauss function enables reading the probability value of meeting a given, selected by us, value of the feature measured (which is shown in Fig. 2.3.). In that case we find the value $x$, that we are interested in (e.g. a person of 48), and then we read the probability corresponding to that value.

---

[18] The research connected with the norm definition, which is to say the value accepted as the result corresponding to a healthy person condition, is constantly conducted in medical sciences. Constant monitoring of the population of the healthy people population inhabiting e.g. the given country is indispensable with respect to the constantly changing living conditions, nutrition habits, the stress factors, etc.

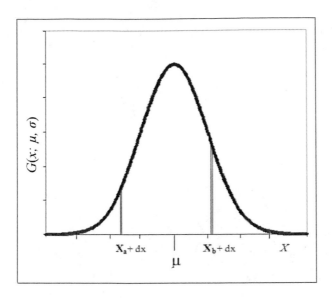

**Fig. 2.4.** The way of reading the probability values ($p_a$, $p_b$) for the assigned values $x_a$ and $x_b$. which are really the probabilities to find the values for intervals ($x_a + dx$) and ($x_b + dx$) where $dx$ represents arbitrarily small range

From the normal distribution, we can also read the range probability value of meeting the result from the given number range (Fig. 2.4.).

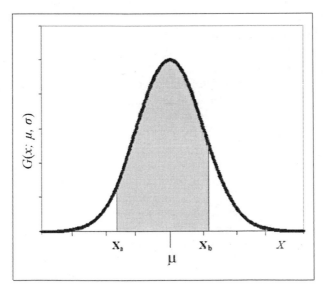

**Fig. 2.5.** The range probability – the probability of meeting $X$ values from the range $x_a$ to $x_b$ is graphically expressed with the area size in proportion to the whole area between the function graph line and the $X$-axis. Mathematically, that area surface signifies the sum (integral) of appearance probabilities of the values from the given range

The interest range selection is arbitrary, which is also shown in Fig. 2.5.

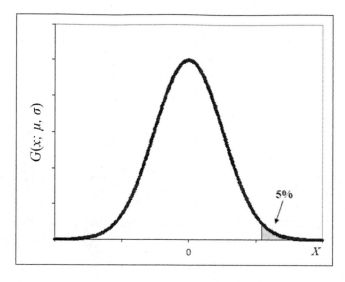

**Fig. 2.6.** The range probability for the high levels of $X$ values that constitute 5% of the $X$ values

Fig. 2.6. presents the area that represents the probability value of meeting the measurement results from the range marked grey. The point on $X$-axis specific to the grey area presents the value that delimits 5% of all the values, but simultaneously those values are the highest values in the group.

Thus, we can read the probability of meeting a person of the assigned age, or a person who belongs to the appointed age range. The condition is the fact, though, that the given measurable feature distribution observed in the analysed sample represents normal distribution. It can prove, though, that despite such expectations, the measured value distribution does not represent such a distribution.

One more notion connected with the issues concerning the distribution is important. The *normal standardised distribution* – in order to explain this notion, it is necessary to learn a very simple mathematical transformation, which transforms any normal distribution. This will be explained using an example. Fig. 2.6. presents the (theoretical) distribution probability of the given calcium compounds concentration emerging in the nephrolithiasis patient's urine. In one group there are women (the black line), in whom additionally osteoporosis was found, in the other group there are women with nephrolithiasis in whom no osteoporosis was found (the green line).

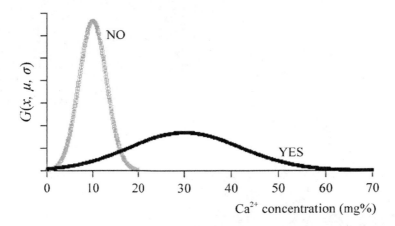

**Fig. 2.7.** Distribution values of calcium ion concentration in the patients' urine in two groups: of those with osteoporosis found (YES), and those in whom that illness was not found (NO)

In the illustrations, it is easy to localize arithmetic mean values and standard deviation values. It is clearly visible that these charts differ from each other with their situation on the $X$-axis (other arithmetic mean values) and the dispersion level (measured with standard deviation value). Is it possible to compare the two distributions? If we imagine that analogous charts were obtained by other researchers engaged in similar issues, the variety of those charts is likely to cause that comparing them is more and more complex. The solution is normal distribution standardization, which consists in a very simple procedure:

$$Z = \frac{x - \mu}{\sigma}$$ (eq. 2.13.)

$$Z_i = \frac{x_i - \bar{x}}{s}$$ (eq. 2.14.)

We introduced the new variable $Z$, which is directly connected to the primary variable $X$, and also contains all those values that specified the primary variable distribution $N(\bar{x}, s)$.

We shall interpret the essence of the suggested operation by means of the following illustration:

Let us draw a new axis of $Z$-variable parallel to the $X$-line.

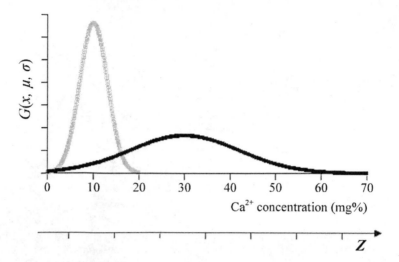

**Fig. 2.8.** The new axis relation for the standardized variable Z

The first question is: What value will appear on the Z-axis in the analogous place to the position of $\bar{x}$ values on the X-axis? In the place analogous to $\bar{x}$ on the Z-axis, the value of 0.0 will appear, which results from the simple calculation of the Z value, after substituting the arithmetic mean $\bar{x}$ in place of $x_i$ (Fig. 2.8.).

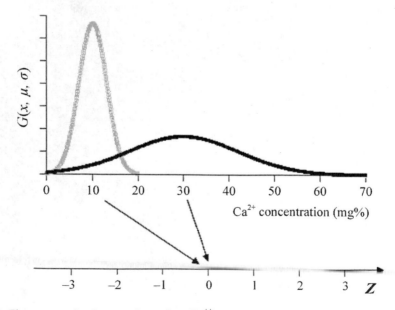

**Fig. 2.9.** The measured value transformation ($Ca^{++}$ concentration in mg%) to the Z variable scale

The measured feature value, to which the maximum probability corresponds, is situated in the 0 position on Z-axis after the transformation (Fig. 2.9.).

The second question is: What value on the Z-axis corresponds to the position of $\bar{x} + s$ on the X-axis? Again, a simple calculation says, that the value is 1.
In the same way, in place of $\bar{x} - s$ on the Z-axis the value of $-1$ will appear (Fig. 2.10.).

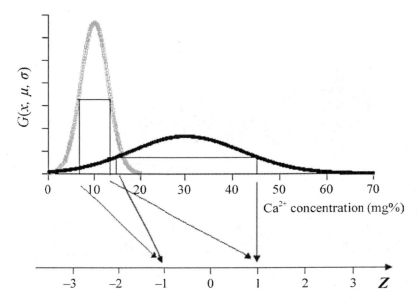

**Fig. 2.10.** The measured feature transformation ($Ca^{++}$ concentration in mg%) to the scale of Z variable.

The value of the feature measured corresponding to $\bar{x} - s$ and $\bar{x} + s$ is situated in the positions $-1$ and 1 respectively on the Z-axis after the transformation.

The further analysis: Let assume, that the measurement variable in the analysed example was the calcium salts concentration in the female patients' urine. The unit that expresses it is mg%.
Another question is: What measure does the new variable Z represent?
Analysing the formula structure we can see, that Z is a measureless value.
On the X-axis, if we move by a measure unit (1 mg%), it signifies the increase of calcium salts concentration by one mg%. What does moving by 1 on the Z-axis signify?
It proves, that the unit on the Z-axis is one standard deviation value regardless its value in the X-scale. We can see that the value $\bar{x}_{with} - s_{with}$ for the women with osteoporosis and the value $\bar{x}_{without} - s_{without}$ for the women without osteoporosis have met in the same place on the Z-axis. So we can see, that irrespectively of the value of standard deviation calculated for the measured feature, those points (and the values represented by them) meet in the appropriate places on the new Z-axis.

If we generalize our procedure to any charts of the distribution probability, regardless what feature they represent and what parameters $(\bar{x}, s)$ were calculated for them, the charts meet in the standardized arrangement. In other words, if all the possible distributions $N(\bar{x}, s)$ of any $\bar{x}$ and $s$ values were standardized, they would meet in one common place. What is more, they would cover each other giving one chart that is called the *normal standardized distribution*. The Reader will not be surprised that the notation of such distribution is $N(0,1)$. The mean for the standardized distribution is 0, and the standard deviation value is 1. Number 1 in the normal distribution notation signifies the value that differs by one from the arithmetic mean (that in this case equals 0) (Fig. 2.11.). What "by one" means, is that it differs by the value of one standard deviation (which really amounts as much as it was calculated for particular measurable variable).

The consequence of this operation is the fact, that in such a situation there can be an unlimited number of normal distributions, the normal standardized distribution is only one. To some extent, it is a matrix or a template according to which we can estimate all the other empirical distributions that have ever appeared in our empirical analysis.

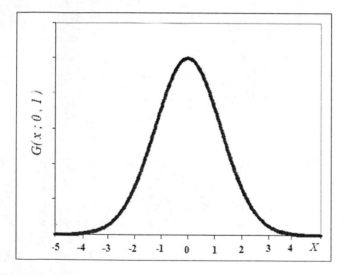

**Fig. 2.11.** The normal standardized distribution chart. The arithmetic mean read for the maximum probability equals 0 and the standard deviation equals 1

There is one more consequence of the fact that there is one standardized normal distribution. We can read the function values for this distribution from one table, common for all users. Those values constitute a certain universal standard. In the age of computers, we can calculate the function values for any $Z$ value any time. It is also important that performing the operation reverse to the one given above, we can calculate any time the value of the feature being measured ($X$) that corresponds to the given value of the variable $Z$.

Operations of this type will be used in order to determine the so-called *confidence range* and to assign the so-called minimum number for the representative sample. As it has already been said, the number of cases analysed in a given sample is of extreme importance if we plan generalizing the results obtained to the whole population. It is connected with the fact of not admitting operating upon the data whose number of freedom degrees approaches zero, what makes impossible the generalization of the results obtained to other patients' groups, not included in the analysed group. The objective of using statistics, which is the possibility of generalizing to the whole population the results obtained on the basis of the sample analysis, would be unattainable then.

It is also worthwhile to turn attention to another feature connected to the transition from the theoretical distribution to the normal (empirical) distribution. The basic difference consists in the number of cases to support the distribution analysis. The theoretical distribution for the population defines the relation for the unlimited number of the $x$ variable values while the sample contains finite number of elements. The consequence of this is the fact, that each empirical distribution can be expressed with the accuracy up to the measured values range. That problem was signalled when the measurable feature character was specified as continuous, while each measurable feature must be really treated as abrupt because of the limited measurement accuracy. Hence, the empirical distribution always assumes the bar diagram shape, as it was shown in Fig. 2.12.

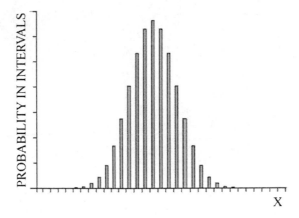

**Fig. 2.12.** The empirical distribution characterizing only the range probability (for the finite number of elements in the sample and for the finite measurement accuracy)

The empirical distribution, represented with the range probability values, can be compared to the theoretical distribution when the probability value for the theoretical distribution has been calculated (already discussed probability values addition rule).

A comparison of the theoretical distribution to the empirical distribution for the analysed sample of the patients with the renal colic in the group of men and women (the calculation details in the workbook part) is presented in the illustrations below:

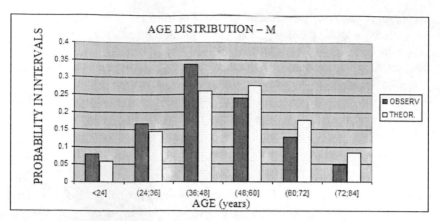

**Fig. 2.13.** The empirical distribution of the patients' age in the sample of male patients with nephrolithiasis (the dark histogram) in comparison to the theoretical distribution (the light histogram). The empirical distribution can assume only the histogram form (the range probability), as the sample always contains a finite number of measurements. The illustration enables the empirical (observed in our sample) distribution comparison in relation to the theoretical (expected) distribution, so it could be presented in the form of an unbroken line. Because of a clear exposure of the differences, the theoretical distribution was also presented in the form of a histogram

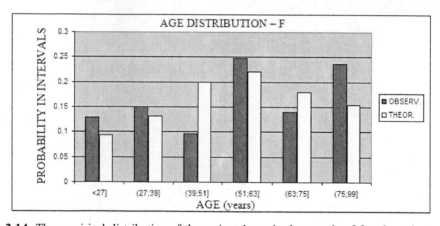

**Fig. 2.14.** The empirical distribution of the patients' age in the sample of female patients with nephrolithiasis (the dark histogram) compared to the theoretical distribution (the light histogram). The empirical distribution can assume only the histogram form (range probability), as the sample always contains a finite number of measurements. The illustration enables the comparison of the empirical distribution (observed in our sample) in relation to the theoretical (expected) distribution that could be presented as the unbroken line. Because of a clear exposure of the differences, the theoretical distribution was also presented in the form of a histogram. Our analysis series we enabled to estimate the male and female nephrolithiasis patients' age analysis. On the basis of the distribution obtained the empirical distribution of the age group. Comparing the empirical distribution and the theoretical (expected) distribution enables formulating a statement (for the time being subjectively), that there are certain differences between the theoretical distribution and the age distribution among the male and female patients. The male patients' age distribution seems to be closer to the theoretical (expected) distribution than in the case of women

The objective of our further analysis will be the finding if our subjective estimation is confirmed by the application of the statistical tests that objectively state the presence (or absence) of differences between the theoretical (normal) distribution and the empirical distribution (observed in our group of patients).

## Exercises

1. Choose one measurable feature thematically connected with the issue formulated at the point? I.2. and copy it to the new spreadsheet.
2. Put the values of a chosen feature in the ascending order.
3. Perform all the operations according to the example presented in this chapter (see exercise part).
4. Present graphically the range and the accumulated probability distribution both for the theoretical and the empirical distribution.
5. Describe the conclusions resulting from confronting both graphic forms of the results presentation.
6. Estimate subjectively the value of the differences between the empirical and the theoretical distribution. Do you think that the differences between the theoretical distribution and the empirical distribution are negligible or do you think that they are essential, so it is eventually impossible to determine if /that the empirical distribution can be specified as compliant with the theoretical distribution?
7. Revise all the analysis separately for the group of people who survived and for those who did not survive the traffic accident (filling in the appropriate people sets to the separate spreadsheets).

# STEP 2 – exercise

# Data analysis

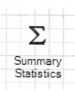

Summary
Statistics

In this step we learn how to determine the empirical distribution and corresponding theoretical distribution (parameters: arithmetic mean and standard deviation in accordance with the previous calculations). Plots will show us a subjective difference between the distributions.

In this example we use Excel sheets to follow the procedures in the SAS package by selecting options. By performing all steps in a single calculation the reader will find out that the statistical procedure is not a magic secret. All operations can be applied by a person without specialist knowledge.

1. Our list of data (column A – age of patients) should be sorted (for instance in ascending order – column B).

| | A | B |
|---|---|---|
| | AGE - M | AGE - M |
| 1 | | |
| 2 | 21 | 2 |
| 3 | 48 | 4 |
| 4 | 54 | 8 |
| 5 | 56 | 11 |
| 6 | 72 | 14 |
| 7 | 44 | 15 |
| 8 | 48 | 16 |
| 9 | 49 | 18 |
| 10 | 51 | 19 |
| 11 | 50 | 20 |
| 12 | 26 | 21 |

**Fig. 2.1.** Part of the table with the ages of patients. Column A presents the data in chronological order whereas Column B in an ordered array from the smallest value to the largest value

2. Determine the minimal and maximal value in our column (cells D2, D3).
3. Compute the arithmetic mean and the standard deviation (cells D5, D6).

|   | A | B | C | D |
|---|---|---|---|---|
| 1 | AGE - M | AGE - M | | |
| 2 | 21 | 2 | MIN | 2 |
| 3 | 48 | 4 | MAX | 97 |
| 4 | 54 | 8 | | |
| 5 | 56 | 11 | AVERAGE | 49.5 |
| 6 | 72 | 14 | ST.DEV. | 16.31 |
| 7 | 44 | 15 | | |

**Fig. 2.2.** Basic descriptive data: the minimum, the maximum, the arithmetic mean and the standard deviation

4. The minimal and maximal values facilitate the determination of the intervals that make sense in the case of our variable. Class intervals for a given dataset may be specified by using a formula given by Sturges for the number of class intervals. This formula gives (cell D8):

$$LK = 1 + 3.222 \log n ,$$

where $n$ stands for the number of values in the dataset under consideration.

| $f_x$ =1+3.222*LOG10(163) | | |
|---|---|---|
| C | D | E |
| | | |
| MIN | 2 | |
| MAX | 97 | |
| | | |
| AVERAGE | 49.5 | |
| ST.DEV. | 16.31 | |
| | | |
| | | |
| | | |
| LK | 8.127668 | |

**Fig. 2.3.** More parameters appear in the spreadsheet. The number of classes (LK) has been added by applying the formula on the formula bar

5. Based of the number of class intervals we calculate the smallest and the largest value for these intervals (cells F2... F10 – Fig. 2.5.):
A – To this purpose R (the range) (D7) is divided by the number of classes (LK – the value rounded down) we desire to group our set of observations (Fig. 2.4. position D 11).

$$P_{rz} = \frac{R}{LK}$$

| D11 | ▼ | $f_x$ =D7/8 | |
|---|---|---|---|

| | A | B | C | D |
|---|---|---|---|---|
| 1 | AGE - M | AGE - M | | |
| 2 | 21 | 2 | MIN | 2 |
| 3 | 48 | 4 | MAX | 97 |
| 4 | 54 | 8 | | |
| 5 | 56 | 11 | AVERAGE | 49.5 |
| 6 | 72 | 14 | ST.DEV. | 16.31 |
| 7 | 44 | 15 | RANGE | 95 |
| 8 | 48 | 16 | | |
| 9 | 49 | 18 | | |
| 10 | 51 | 19 | LK | 8.127668 |
| 11 | 50 | 20 | CLASS | 11.875 |

**Fig. 2.4.** Additionally we have determined the width of the class interval (by applying the formula on the formula bar) for men

B – We construct our intervals, by adding one, two, three and more class intervals to the smallest value. As a result we obtain our intervals as shown in Column F (Fig. 2.5.). Note the parentheses. The parenthesis „(„ marks the extreme value excluded whereas „]" marks the extreme value included in the interval. For this reason 12 does not fall within the second class interval but falls in the first class interval.

| | A | B | C | D | E | F |
|---|---|---|---|---|---|---|
| 1 | AGE - M | AGE - M | | | | CLASS |
| 2 | 21 | 2 | MIN | 2 | | (0;12] |
| 3 | 48 | 4 | MAX | 97 | | (12;24] |
| 4 | 54 | 8 | | | | (24;36] |
| 5 | 56 | 11 | AVERAGE | 49.5 | | (36;48] |
| 6 | 72 | 14 | ST.DEV. | 16.31 | | (48;60] |
| 7 | 44 | 15 | RANGE | 95 | | (60;72] |
| 8 | 48 | 16 | | | | (72;84] |
| 9 | 49 | 18 | | | | (84;96] |
| 10 | 51 | 19 | LK | 8.13 | | (96;108] |
| 11 | 50 | 20 | CLASS | 11.87 | | |
| 12 | 26 | 21 | | | | |

**Fig. 2.5.** Column F contains class interval ranges. The opening parenthesis „(„ marks the value that does not fall within the class interval and the closing bracket „]" marks the value that falls within the interval for men

The problem is the minimal value, which – in accordance with the notation – should not fall within class interval 1. In this case (in the case of class 1) we make an exception and enlarge this interval starting with 0.

6. Another step is to determine the number of observations (subjects) falling within the first, second, third etc. class interval.

We use Excel and the standard "COUNTIF" function. The value equal to or smaller than the upper limit in the class interval is the condition to be met in counting (Fig. 2.6.).

| $f_x$ =COUNTIF(B2:B164;<12.1) | | | | | | | | | |
|---|---|---|---|---|---|---|---|---|---|
| C | D | E | F | G | H | I | J | K | L |
| | | | CLASS | | | | | | |
| MIN | 2 | | (0;12] | I;<12.1) | | | | | |
| MAX | 97 | | (12;24] | | | | | | |
| | | | (24;36] | **Function Arguments** | | | | | |
| AVERAGE | 49.5 | | (36;48] | COUNTIF | | | | | |
| ST.DEV. | 16.31 | | (48;60] | Range B2:B164 | | = | | | |
| RANGE | 95 | | (60;72] | Criteria <12.1 | | = | | | |
| | | | (72;84] | | | | | | |
| | | | (84;96] | | | = | | | |
| LK | 8.13 | | (96;108] | Counts the number of cells within a range that meet the given condition. | | | | | |
| CLASS | 11.87 | | | | | | | | |

**Fig. 2.6.** The way of counting subjects within a given class interval in the cumulative form for men

7. We obtain the *cumulative frequency* of values (Fig. 2.7.). The number of subjects 40 within the third class interval denotes the number of subjects with the observations (ages) smaller than or equal to 36, i.e. it denotes the number of all subjects falling within the first, second and third class interval. For this reason it is called the cumulative frequency.

| C | G |
|---|---|
| CLASS | CUMMUL. |
| (0;12] | 4 |
| (12;24] | 14 |
| (24;36] | 40 |
| (36;48] | 95 |
| (48;60] | 134 |
| (60;72] | 155 |
| (72;84] | 161 |
| (84;96] | 162 |
| (96;108] | 163 |

**Fig. 2.7.** Cumulative frequencies obtained within all class intervals for men

8. Frequencies within each class interval are obtained by subtracting from the cumulative frequency the cumulative frequency of the previous class interval (Fig. 2.8.).

| fx | =D4-D3 | |
|---|---|---|

| C | D | E |
|---|---|---|
| **CLASS** | **CUMMUL.** | **NUMB.** |
| (0;12] | 4 | 4 |
| (12;24] | 14 | 10 |
| (24;36] | 40 | 26 |
| (36;48] | 95 | |
| (48;60] | 134 | |
| (60;72] | 155 | |
| (72;84] | 161 | |
| (84;96] | 162 | |
| (96;108] | 163 | |

| C | D | E |
|---|---|---|
| **CLASS** | **CUMMUL.** | **NUMB.** |
| (0;12] | 4 | 4 |
| (12;24] | 14 | 10 |
| (24;36] | 40 | 26 |
| (36;48] | 95 | 55 |
| (48;60] | 134 | 39 |
| (60;72] | 155 | 21 |
| (72;84] | 161 | 6 |
| (84;96] | 162 | 1 |
| (96;108] | 163 | 1 |

**Fig. 2.8.** Cumulative frequencies calculated for frequencies within each class interval for men

If absolute frequencies are represented as a fraction, we obtain the empirical probability (resulting from our study) of occurrence of the data element that falls within a given class interval. We accomplish this by dividing all frequencies within class intervals by the total number of subjects (elements) in the dataset under consideration.

9. If we choose from a long list of graphic displays, we obtain the following distributions:
   A – cumulative probability distribution,
   B – probability of occurrence of a value that falls within a given class.

| | G10 | ▼ | | *fx* =E10/163 | | |
|---|---|---|---|---|---|---|
| | A | B | C | D | E | F | G |
| 1 | AGE - M | AGE - M | CLASS | CUMMUL. | NUMB. | CUMM.PROB. | PROBABILITY |
| 2 | 21 | 2 | (0;12] | 4 | 4 | 0.024539877 | 0.024539877 |
| 3 | 48 | 4 | (12;24] | 14 | 10 | 0.085889571 | 0.061349693 |
| 4 | 54 | 8 | (24;36] | 40 | 26 | 0.245398773 | 0.159509202 |
| 5 | 56 | 11 | (36;48] | 95 | 55 | 0.582822086 | 0.337423313 |
| 6 | 72 | 14 | (48;60] | 134 | 39 | 0.82208589 | 0.239263804 |
| 7 | 44 | 15 | (60;72] | 155 | 21 | 0.950920245 | 0.128834356 |
| 8 | 48 | 16 | (72;84] | 161 | 6 | 0.987730061 | 0.036809816 |
| 9 | 49 | 18 | (84;96] | 162 | 1 | 0.993865031 | 0.006134969 |
| 10 | 51 | 19 | (96;108] | 163 | 1 | 1 | 0.006134969 |
| 11 | 50 | 20 | | | | TOTAL | 1 |

**Fig. 2.9.** Table of frequencies including cumulative probability (Column F) and probability within class intervals (Column G) for men

The term cumulative probability is quite simple. It shows the probability that the random variable will attain a value less than or equal to each value that the random variable can take on. If the cutoff value is 48, the probability that a subject is 48 years old or younger is 0.55. By determining a cutoff value that is important to us, we obtain more information about our dataset. For instance, if we want to know the probability of occurrence of juveniles in our dataset, we ask about the probability of occurrence of a subject 18 years old or younger. The cumulative probability distribution is used in practice to determine the half probability.

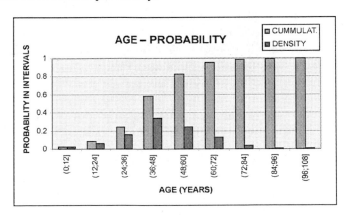

**Fig. 2.10.** Cumulative frequency distribution (light bars) and frequencies within class intervals (dark bars) for men

The graph shows the value of the measurement which cuts off half of the group with low measurements (age group 4). We may also ask which value identifies subjects (on the *X*-axis) who make up 1/3 or any other proportion of the dataset.

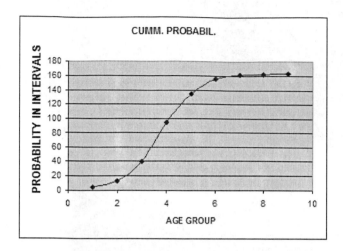

**Fig. 2.11.** Cumulative probability plot. The *X*-axis shows only the numbers corresponding to class intervals. The *Y*-axis shows cumulative probability values. The cumulative probability is about 1. The probability of occurrence of the value equal to or less than the maximal value can be predicted with certainty that is with probability equal to unity (according to Column D Fig. 2.8.)

The cumulative distribution function rises asymptotically to unity. In the empirical distributions the cumulative distribution function equal to unity is obtained for the largest measurement in our dataset (the oldest subject).

The reason why we constructed this distribution is to find out whether it differs from the normal or Gaussian distribution. The theoretical distribution may be converted into class intervals, calculating the sum of probabilities for each class interval defined. By comparing the theoretical and empirical distribution we may assess differences between the expected and genuine distribution (relative to a given measurable characteristic).

The theoretical distribution fitting a Gaussian distribution can be constructed using the function plot. We should know the value of two parameters only: the mean and standard deviation (calculated for our dataset).

Without going into details, the procedure is as follows (Fig. 2.12.):

1. In Column I we enter upper class limits.
2. In Column J, after positioning the cursor as shown below, we select the NORMDIST function from the pop-up menu.
3. In the window that appears we are asked to provide the cell reference of the arithmetic mean and standard deviation. In the last window we enter the word TRUE.

$f_x$ =NORMDIST(I2;$D$12;$D$13;TRUE)

| C | D | E | F | G | H | I | J |
|---|---|---|---|---|---|---|---|
| CLASS | CUMMUL. | NUMB. | CUMM.PROB. | PROBABILITY | CLASS | UPPER LIMIT | T.C.PR. |
| (0;12] | 4 | 4 | 0.024539877 | 0.024539877 | (0;12] | 12 | };TRUE) |
| (12;24] | 14 | 10 | 0.085889571 | 0.061349693 | (12;24] | 24 | |
| (24;36] | 40 | 26 | 0.245398773 | 0.159509202 | (24;36] | 36 | |
| (36;48] | 95 | | | | | | |
| (48;60] | 134 | | | | | | |
| (60;72] | 155 | | | | | | |
| (72;84] | 161 | | | | | | |
| (84;96] | 162 | | | | | | |
| (96;108] | 163 | | | | | | |
| AVER | 49.5 | | | | | | |
| ST.DEV. | 16.31 | | | | | | |

**Function Arguments** ✕

NORMDIST

| | | |
|---|---|---|
| X | I2 | = 12 |
| Mean | $D$12 | = 49.5 |
| Standard_dev | $D$13 | = 16.31 |
| Cumulative | TRUE | = TRUE |

**Fig. 2.12.** Construction of the theoretical (fitting a Gaussian distribution) cumulative probability

4. Spreading the formula to all the cells in the column brings up the cumulative probability (in accordance with the instructions in the lower part of the dialog box).

| CLASS | T.C.PR. | THEOR.PROB. |
|---|---|---|
| (0;12] | 0.010747 | 0.010746709 |
| (12;24] | 0.058972 | 0.048225744 |
| (24;36] | 0.203917 | 0.144944057 |
| (36;48] | 0.463362 | 0.259445175 |
| (48;60] | 0.74014 | 0.276778232 |
| (60;72] | 0.916133 | 0.175993112 |
| (72;84] | 0.982796 | 0.066663359 |
| (84;96] | 0.997821 | 0.015024593 |
| (96;108] | 0.999833 | 0.00201161 |
| TOTAL | | 0.999832592 |

**Fig. 2.13.** Theoretical cumulative distributions and the probabilities calculated within class intervals for men

5. By repeating the previous procedure to replace the cumulative probability with the group probability scale (for classes) we obtain a new column containing the probabilities within the class intervals.
6. By selecting the bar chart to present the values and by highlighting Column show THEOR. PROB. in Fig.2.13. we obtain a graph as shown in Fig. 2.14.

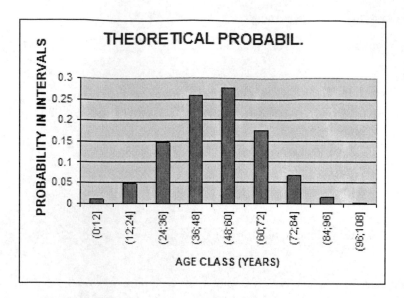

**Fig. 2.14.** Theoretical probability distribution. The *X*-axis represents age classes. The *Y*-axis provides the probability values fitting a Gaussian distribution for men

7. By selecting the columns with the empirical and theoretical probability, we can view both distributions in one table. It is possible because age ranges are the same for both data (observed and theoretical).

| CLASS | THEOR.PROB. | OBS.PROB. |
|---|---|---|
| (0;12] | 0.010746709 | 0.024539877 |
| (12;24] | 0.048225744 | 0.061349693 |
| (24;36] | 0.144944057 | 0.159509202 |
| (36;48] | 0.259445175 | 0.337423313 |
| (48;60] | 0.276778232 | 0.239263804 |
| (60;72] | 0.175993112 | 0.128834356 |
| (72;84] | 0.066663359 | 0.036809816 |
| (84;96] | 0.015024593 | 0.006134969 |
| (96;108] | 0.00201161 | 0.006134969 |
| TOTAL | 0.999832592 | 1 |

**Fig. 2.15.** Observed and theoretical probability distribution within the age class intervals for men

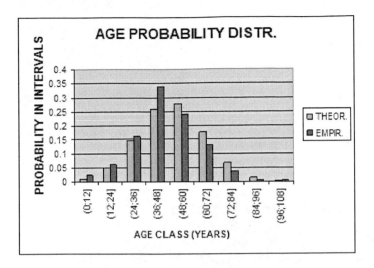

**Fig. 2.16.** Histogram of the data with the observed (constructed from patient data) and theoretical (fitting a Gaussian distribution) distributions for men

8. The same operation on columns with the cumulative values (empirical and theoretical) will facilitate the presentation of our results in another form i.e. the cumulative probability distribution where the theoretical and empirical distribution is compared. This time the Gaussian distribution is similar to the sigmoid curve which is also a symmetrical double curve, whereas the Gaussian function curve is the mirror symmetrical curve.

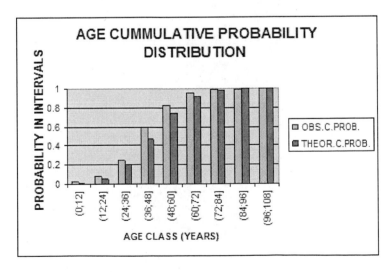

**Fig. 2.17.** Histogram of the observed probability distribution (light) and histogram of the theoretical probability distribution (dark) for men

Remember that the cumulative probability is the probability of a result less than or equal to $(x_0)$.

$$P_c(x_0) = P(x \leq x_0)$$

If we sum all the probabilities for a given dataset, it will be equal to unity. What does it mean? It means that the probability of any result to occur between the MIN and MAX value is a certainty. In the formula expressing the probability definition (see the eq. 2.2. in STEP 2 of theoretical part of this manual) m = n denotes that each random selection of the value between the MIN and MAX is satisfactory and thus probability is certainty.

If we perform an identical analysis for women we obtain a table as shown below.

| CLASSES | NUMBERS | PR. OBS. | P. THEOR. |
|---------|---------|----------|-----------|
| (3;15]  | 3       | 0.0322   | 0.0298    |
| (15;27] | 7       | 0.0752   | 0.0638    |
| (27;39] | 17      | 0.1829   | 0.1318    |
| (39;51] | 10      | 0.1075   | 0.1996    |
| (51;63] | 20      | 0.215    | 0.2214    |
| (63;75] | 15      | 0.1613   | 0.1801    |
| (75;87] | 19      | 0.2043   | 0.1073    |
| (87;99] | 2       | 0.0215   | 0.0468    |
| TOTAL   | 93      | 0.9999   | 0.9806    |

**Fig. 2.18.** Frequency distribution, observed and theoretical probabilities for women

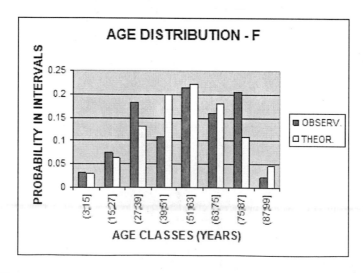

**Fig. 2.19.** Histogram women's age. The observed (dark) and theoretical (white) distribution for women

Our analysis shows the age distribution of male and female patients with nephrolithiasis. When we compare the empirical and theoretical (expected) distributions we find out (subjectively for the time being) that there are some differences in the distribution of ages between males and females. At first sight the age distribution of men is closer to the theoretical (expected) distribution than age distribution of women

The purpose of further analysis is to find out whether our subjective evaluation is confirmed in objective statistical tests for the presence (or absence) of differences between the theoretical (normal) and empirical (observed in our group) distribution.

# STEP 3

# The $\chi^2$ (chi-square) test of the goodness of fit

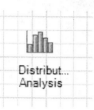

Distribut...
Analysis

**Is the women's age distribution (in the group of people with the urinary tract nephrolithiasis) a normal distribution?**
**Is the men's age distribution (in the group of people with the urinary tract nephrolithiasis) a normal distribution?**

We hope that a careful Reader has already noticed the importance of stating if the analysed feature (age) meets the conditions of normal distribution. We can estimate it subjectively, of course, analysing e.g. two distributions (the empirical and the theoretical one, presented in Fig 2.16. and 2.19.). If our decision is to be objective, let us use the instrument, which is the statistical test that enables **objectivization** of such a decision.

Before we learn the statistical test, let us specify the notion of the *testing procedure*. The *testing procedure* is a set of certain operations, which, performed in the right sequence and under specified conditions, constitute exactly the universal instrument of statistical analysis. Especially the statistical test enables making an objective decision (with some level of probability of an error) concerning a certain phenomenon. The decision is expressed with stating the possibility of rejection (or no reason to reject) a certain statement that specifies the presence or absence of a certain statement that determines the significance or insignificance of differences between certain parameters. In our case, we are going to study the significance of differences between the empirical and the theoretical distribution.

It has been stated that testing statistical hypotheses is a certain performance instruction. The instruction consists of the specific steps:

1. We must ask a detailed question concerning the issue currently discussed – in our case the question concerns the differences between the theoretical and empirical distribution. The analysis objective is determining if the negligence of the existing differences would not be a major error. In the contrary case we shall state that the difference is essential. The statement that we want to assume as true is called the *null hypothesis*, signified as $H_0$. Usually, the statement contained in $H_0$ has the form of the negative sentence that ignores the differences. Specifically, in our example, the $H_0$ sounds:

"There is no difference between the empirical and the theoretical (normal) distribution".

As this sentence is not going to prove true for all the cases, we also define the *alternative hypothesis* $H_1$. Its substance is a negation of the statement expressed in $H_0$. In our example, $H_1$ says:

"There is a difference between the empirical and the theoretical distribution".

2. We also said that we wanted our decision to bear a possibly objective character. What influences the decision objectivity?

A – In the statistics, one of the essential elements of objectivism is the number of cases analysed in the given research project.
The larger the sample, the higher the share of objectivism in our research. The influence of the number of elements in the sample for the objectivity is not given directly. It is expressed with the *number freedom degrees*. The higher the number of degrees of freedom the higher the chance for our decision to have a really objective character which is to say that other, independent researchers confirm our observations. If the sample is not large enough, the possibility of the confirmation absence for our observation in a study conducted by another researcher becomes more probable. The number of degrees of freedom is calculated in the way that is specific for a given test. In case of our analysis of differences between the distributions, we calculate it in the following way:

$$df = LK - 1, \qquad \text{(eq. 3.1.)}$$

where $df$ signifies the number of degrees of freedom, $LK$ signifies the number of classes into which the primary data set was divided (the number of classes, as it was shown in the workbook part, strictly follows the sample's size).

B – The second structural element of the objectivism of our decision is the awareness and compliance to the risk of committing a certain error, as we shall never analyse all the cases (the population is not accessible for studies). The sample choice always bears the risk of committing an error when making a decision concerning the differences between the distributions (or any other decision). The awareness of a possibility of committing an error and the acceptance of a certain level of the error is expressed in assuming the so-called *significance level*. The significance level (usually expressed in percent – %) signifies, that we agree to the fact, that we can make wrong decision but the probability of it is less than assumed level. Usually the significance level is assumed as 5% (frequently denoted as 0.05). The level, assumed by a researcher, is to be a certain consensus between the expectations (the minimum possible error risk) and the awareness of the data imperfection.

If the test will be then conducted on the basis of the subjective data (the patient himself/herself estimates his/her health condition or the habits, etc.), that can *a priori* bear a serious error, we must not impose very rigorous requirements and assume a very low significance level opposite to the studies of high objectiveness degree, e.g. based upon the measurable data and automatically conducted with the specialist laboratory equipment.

Besides, the awareness of the consequences of our study is also important. If we conduct it in training purposes or as an entertainment (e.g. to verify the beauty contest results), the assumed level can be higher, e.g. 10%. But, in case of e.g. testing a new compound that we assume to be a medical drug, and the consequence of our decision is the responsibility for introducing it to the drug stores and general application, we must not allow ourselves for too high significance level, which is to say too high risk of error committing.[19]

In such cases the level of 1%, and even of 0.1% is appropriate.

The significance level should be **assumed (by the researcher) at the very beginning of the test** and should be an expression of the aware and critical estimate of the importance and meaning of the given analysis.

In our example we shall assume the significance level that equals 5%.

3. Coming back to the basic question about the significance of the differences between the distributions one can see that the answer to this question depends on what we assume as the comparison criterion. I do not think to surprise many readers saying that the criterion in our example is just a sum of differences between the heights of the columns that represent probability values in particular intervals (bar chart – histogram). However, if we calculated the sum of differences it could prove to be zero, at considerable differences of the columns' height. It could result from the fact that sometimes that difference would have the plus (+) mark, and sometimes the minus (–) mark. In order to avoid this confusion, the sum of second power of all differences (in classes) is calculated. In order to make the quantitative result still more universal, the differences are expressed in relative form (the squares of the differences between the empirical probability and the theoretical probability values divided by the theoretical

---

[19] In the further part of the book the notion of the significance level will be explained in a detailed way.

probability values). The way of calculating the quantitative value of the differences estimation criterion is expressed with the formula:

$$\chi^2 = \sum_{i=1}^{r} \frac{(n_i - np_i)^2}{np_i} \qquad \text{(eq. 3.2.)}$$

$$\chi^2 = n\sum_{i=1}^{r} \frac{(p_{ti} - p_{ei})^2}{p_{ti}}, \qquad \text{(eq. 3.3.)}$$

where:  $n$ – total size (total number of observations),
$n_i$ – size observed in the $i$-th class (number of observations in the $i$-th class),
$p_i$ – probability of meeting the result in the $i$-class,
index $e$ signifies – empirical, $t$ – theoretical,
$r$ – the number of ranges (classes).

The two versions of the formula (eq. 3.2. and eq. 3.3.) express exactly the same value (one form can be transduced into another). The expression that was described verbally above is the formula introduced as the second one.

Calculating the numerical value expressing the differences between the theoretical and empirical distribution for our men and women group are illustrated in Fig. 3.1.

| CLASSES | NUMBER | PR. OBS. | PR. THEOR. |
|---------|--------|----------|------------|
| (3;15]  | 3      | 0.0322   | 0.0298     |
| (15;27] | 7      | 0.0752   | 0.0638     |
| (27;39] | 17     | 0.1828   | 0.1318     |
| (39;51] | 10     | 0.1075   | 0.1996     |
| (51;63] | 20     | 0.215    | 0.2214     |
| (63;75] | 15     | 0.1612   | 0.18       |
| (75;87] | 19     | 0.2043   | 0.1073     |
| (87;99] | 2      | 0.0215   | 0.0468     |
| TOTAL   | 93     | 1        | 0.9805     |

**Fig. 3.1.** The table of values observed and the theoretical range probability values for the age groups with the women patients with nephrolithiasis. The first column (left) represents the class intervals, the second – number of observation in each class, observed probability in the third one followed by the theoretical probability calculated for upper limit of each interval for women

The statistical test $\chi^2$ as many others requires the sample to satisfy some special conditions. The limitation for this test is the number of observation in each class which cannot be lower than 5. To avoid the problem with first class may be incorporated to the second one and last class to the before last.

The final table appropriate for the applicability of $\chi^2$ test is shown in Fig. 3.2.

| | A | B | C | D | E |
|---|---|---|---|---|---|
| 1 | CLASSES | NUMBER | PROB. OBSERV. | PROB. THEORET. | ((PT-PO)^2)/PT |
| 2 | <27] | 12 | 0.1291 | 0.0936 | 0.013464209 |
| 3 | (27;39] | 14 | 0.1505 | 0.1318 | 0.002653187 |
| 4 | (39;51] | 9 | 0.0967 | 0.1996 | 0.053048146 |
| 5 | (51;63] | 23 | 0.2473 | 0.2214 | 0.003029855 |
| 6 | (63;75] | 13 | 0.1398 | 0.1801 | 0.009017712 |
| 7 | (75;99] | 22 | 0.2365 | 0.1541 | 0.04406074 |
| 8 | TOTAL | | 0.9999 | 0.9806 | 0.12527385 |

**Fig. 3.2.** The table shown in Fig. 3.1. after modification. The right column shows the values of the elements the sum calculation according to the formula (eq. 3.2. and 3.3.) for women

4. The calculated value of the differences criterion in the discussed test is 11.642 for women and 10.722 for men. We received values, whose interpretation is still subjective. Is the difference important or negligible? The estimation of the statistics' value (the quantitative difference estimation criterion) takes place at the moment of comparing our calculated statistics of values in relation to the so--called *critical value*.

The *critical value* is likely to be explained using the real life situations. Assume hearing over the radio that the water level in the river has exceeded the critical value we know that the highest acceptable water level must have been exceeded and nobody could underestimate such news. In other words, the water level in the river is on the risk. The critical values of the water in the river are critical for the given area and depend on the land specificity. The critical values for the given test also depend on the values that specify the estimation objectiveness that are the number of degrees of freedom and the significance level. The critical values can be read from the attached table (See Supplement Tables – Tab. S.1.). For that reason the critical value is signified with the test symbol with the α index that expresses the significance level and the *df* that specifies the *degrees of freedom*.

| LEVEL OF SIGNIFICANCE | | | | | |
|---|---|---|---|---|---|
| 0.05 | 0.02 | 0.01 | 0.001 | | |
| 3.841 | 5.412 | 6.635 | 10.827 | 1 | |
| 5.991 | 7.824 | 9.210 | 13.815 | 2 | |
| 7.815 | 9.837 | 11.345 | 16.268 | 3 | |
| 9.488 | 11.668 | 13.277 | 18.465 | 4 | |
| 11.070 | 13.388 | 15.086 | 20.517 | 5 | |
| 12.592 | 15.033 | 16.812 | 22.457 | 6 | |
| 14.067 | 16.622 | 18.475 | 24.322 | 7 | |
| 15.507 | 18.168 | 20.090 | 26.125 | 8 | |
| 16.919 | 19.679 | 21.666 | 27.877 | 9 | |
| 18.307 | 21.161 | 23.209 | 29.588 | 10 | |
| 19.675 | 22.618 | 24.725 | 31.264 | 11 | |
| 21.026 | 24.054 | 26.217 | 32.909 | 12 | |
| 22.362 | 25.472 | 27.688 | 34.528 | 13 | |
| 23.685 | 26.873 | 29.141 | 36.123 | 14 | |
| 24.996 | 28.259 | 30.578 | 37.697 | 15 | |
| 26.296 | 29.633 | 32.000 | 39.252 | 16 | NUMBER OF DEGREES OF FREEDOM |

**Fig. 3.3.** The fragment of the table of the distribution of $\chi^2$ test demonstrating the practical way to find the critical value for $df = 5$ and $\alpha = 5\%$ (See the Tab. S.1.)

5. The critical value for our example (the $\chi^2$ test) of the number of 5 degrees of freedom (6–1) and the significance level of 5% amounts to (the value read from the tables) 11.070 (as shown in Fig. 3.3.)
   The critical values for each statistical test are calculated by the test Author (the distribution of the test statistics). The table of critical values is the integral part of each test. The critical values (as it is easy to notice for a careful Reader, are calculated upon the range probability values, especially with respect to the limit values – as e.g. shown in the Fig. 2.5., while one should remember that the distribution values of statistics can differ from the symmetrical normal distribution, as it was shown in the illustration mentioned).

6. *The final decision.* If the calculated value is above the critical value we must admit that the value of differences exceeded the acceptable level and we must state that the difference analysed by us is statistically relevant and that it is connected with the $H_0$ rejection. However, when the calculated value of the differences is below the critical value, we conclude that there is no reason for the $H_0$ rejection.

Coming back to our example and comparing the relevant values of statistics calculated and critical for the group of men and women (Fig. 3.4.) one should state, that the distribution of the men's age does not differ statistically from the normal distribution, while the age distribution in the group of women is significantly different from the normal distribution.

| F | $\chi^2$ CALCUL. | 11.642 |
|---|---|---|
| DF = 5 | $\chi^2$ CRIT. | 11.070 |
| | | |
| M | $\chi^2$ CALCUL. | 10.722 |
| DF = 5 | $\chi^2$ CRIT. | 11.070 |

**Fig. 3.4.** The table of the $\chi^2$ test calculated value and the critical value for the group of the female and male patients

The final decision concerning the application of the $\chi^2$ accordance test (as it is the name of the test that we have just made) are the following:

In case of men we shall say:

There are no reasons to reject $H_0$, as the value of differences between the distributions (according to the criterion suggested in the $\chi^2$ accordance test) measured with the value of the $\chi^2$ accordance test statistics is higher than the critical value for the men's group, while for the women's group we shall say the following:
$H_0$ must be rejected because the value of the differences between the normal distribution and the empirical distribution (measured with the value of this test statistics) proved to be higher than the critical value.
And that is how we make the final decision that expresses only our attitude towards $H_0$. One should remember that $H_0$ is specific for each test.

7.  INTERPRETATION – As this handbook is addressed to the physicians (medical students) and the whole statistical (and mathematical) details are not of that extreme importance, the way of **interpreting** the final decision that consists in the rejection (or assimilation) of null hypothesis **is totally dependent** upon the physician's responsibility. It is the physician who draws conclusions of medical sense on the basis of statistical analysis.

The medical doctor collaborating with the statistician gets only the information as above – $H_0$ reject or $H_0$ not reject. The medical sense of these sentences is the medical doctor responsibility. This is why the introduction of medical doctors to statistical methods seems to be necessary for fruitful collaboration.

In our example we found out that in case of women the $H_0$ should be rejected, while in case of men we found no reasons for the $H_0$ rejection. It signifies that the age distribution in the group of women is a distribution different from normal and in the same way we cannot apply any normal distribution (function) to represent the empirical distribution. An analogous distribution of the men's age in the analysed group showed that the men's age distribution was a normal distribution.

In general, ascribing the theoretical distribution type to the empirical distribution has plentiful consequences. Firstly, **factually**, we can assume that our expectations with respect to the characteristics of the feature regulated by the natural processes were retained. Secondly, methodologically, we are entitled to perform the mathematical analysis of the distribution parameters if it describes our empirical distribution in the appropriate way. So, all the mathematical operations performed on the function notation can be adapted to the description of our sample and the analysed feature **(e.g. one can assign the scope of the standard)**. That fact influences also the further stages of the complex statistical analysis. There are other tests that we can perform for the variables that represent the normal distribution, and the other for the variables that do not represent them. The mean value when calculated for variable representing the normal distribution expresses the parameter of this distribution. The mean value calculated for two values has nothing common with distribution representation.

Coming back to our patients, in the further part of the handbook we shall try to find out what causes that discrepancy against the expected normal distribution for the group of women. The differences between the women's age distribution related to the men's age distribution will prove medically significant and have a very deep justification.

In that way we have completed the statistical test called the $\chi^2$ *goodness-of-fit test* (called also the accordance test) according to which the significance of differences between the empirical and normal theoretical distribution can be objectively stated.

The *testing procedure* is universal and can apply to many other issues. This universal character of the testing procedure can be expressed with the following generalized instruction:

1. Hypothesis:
   Null hypothesis ($H_0$) – the sentence expressing the fact of ignoring the differences (or the relations) between the comparable groups.
   There is no difference between ........???.....(the further part of $H_0$ is specific for the given test).
   The alternative hypothesis ($H_1$) – a contradiction to $H_0$.
   There is a difference between .......???..(the further part of the hypothesis is specific for the given test).

2. The conditions of the decision objectivity:
   The number of the degrees of freedom *df* – calculated according to the rule obligatory in case of the given test.
   The assumed significance level $\alpha$– accepted by the researcher.

3. The statistics value (the criterion of comparison and the measure of that estimation), calculated with the formula specific to the given test.

4. The critical value – the statistics value assumed in the given case as the liminal value, which is to say dependent on the freedom degrees number and the assumed significance level.

5. The final decision:
If: The statistics value calculated < The critical statistics value – no reason to reject $H_0$.
If: The statistics value calculated > The critical statistics value – $H_0$ is rejected.

6. The interpretation of final results.

The general character of the presented procedure is expressed with the fact, that the arrangement of the particular steps is common for every statistical test, while the exact sound and the way of conducting the calculations (formulae) are specific to the particular tests.
Each of the next tests presented during our course of the basics of statistics follows the procedure presented. The assimilation of such a pattern enables an autonomous activity in the forthcoming part of the course and in future enables autonomous conducting of the correct calculations.

The first of the tests introduced that verified the significance of differences between the theoretical and empirical distribution was the $\chi^2$ accordance test (goodness-of-fit). The test was chosen as the first one for its intuitively clear expression.
There are other tests that verify the differences between the distributions (e.g. Kolmogorov-Smirnov test).[20]

The test is as important as it touches an issue essential to medicine, which is the occurrence of the Gaussian distribution, because (as it has already been told earlier) in relation to all the measurements of the concentrations of the organic fluids components (and other features regulated with the nature laws, including the patient's age) the distribution should appear. If not, it can signify that the variable under consideration may just express a pathological process in discord with the natural rules of regulating the living organism processes. Under such circumstances one should very carefully consider the problem analysed. It can indicate a relevant process, whose disturbance is the object of the medical analysis. A situation should also be excluded, when the feature that constitutes the analysis object underlies a strong influence of an external factor (e.g. applying a medicine that directly influences the examined feature). Finding the essential differences frequently results from the trivial reasons, such as too small size of sample undergoing the analysis. Very often increasing the number of the analysed

---

[20] The Kolmogorov-Smirnov test has an analogous interpretation as the $\chi^2$ test with such a difference that the accumulated probability distribution is the object of the similarity test in target and empirical distribution.

patients influences a better approximation of the empirical distribution to the expected theoretical distribution.

## The outstanding points – The outliers

When analysing the measurable features, it frequently happens to notice the values that considerably depart from the rest of them. A situation like that is presented in the illustration below, where the calcium salts concentration in the patient's urine is shown.

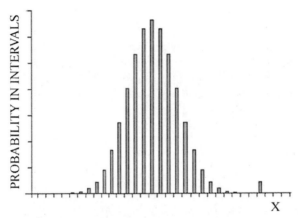

**Fig. 3.5.** The probability distribution demonstrating the so-called outstanding (outliers) points. All the patients represent the values of normal distribution. There is a number of people, though, who differ with the feature measured, representing outstandingly high values

Fig. 3.5. represents the distribution of calcium concentration in urine. As it may be seen the concentration of this ion is very high in small group people in our sample. Such outstanding points may influence significantly the result of the analysis (for example the $\chi^2$ test). This group of people must not be neglected, as it would signify eliminating from the analysis those people, who really exist and who carry essential information concerning the analysed phenomenon. Under such circumstances, it is essential to find out the source of such discrepancy. Anticipating a little our analysis results, we shall satisfy the Reader's curiosity and say that those people are the totally immobilized patients, in whom the process of inappropriate immobilization of calcium from the bones is running, and it is caused by the very immobilization. Those are the people who, apart from the problems connected to the nephrolithiasis, suffer also from multiple sclerosis or are traffic accidents victims with permanent disabilities of central nervous system, or have undergone an intensive chemotherapy in malignant diseases. As visible, they constitute a relatively small group in the sample of people with nephrolithiasis. The moment we identified the cause of so far departed results, we can conduct the further analysis with those people's exclusion. We are entitled to do it by the fact, that we know exactly whom to exclude from the analysis at the given moment. Describing (publishing) the analysis results, each time we inform exactly the reader of our report or a scientific publication of such temporary exclusion of a certain group of patients. It should be pointed out, that in the further part of the analysis we come back to the complete set of people.

Summing up the information concerning the normal distribution, it should be underlined that the characteristic feature of the distribution $N(0,1)$ or $N(\bar{x},s)$ is the equality of all the situation measures of $\bar{x}$, Me and Mo. Mo is one for the normal distribution and equal with respect to the values of the mean $\bar{x}$ and Me. There are also asymmetric distributions of particular skewness, though. The results can prevail whose values are higher against the lower or vice versa. Then we talk about the right- or left-handed distribution (Fig. 3.6.). The diagonality type characteristics can be expressed with the relation between the parameters: $\bar{x}$, Me and Mo.

The measure of the distribution diagonality is the value of kurtosis (kurtosis and skewness) calculated by the majority of programs. The higher the value of kurtosis, the stronger diagonal the analysed distribution is (the kurtosis equal to zero signifies the ideally symmetrical distribution).

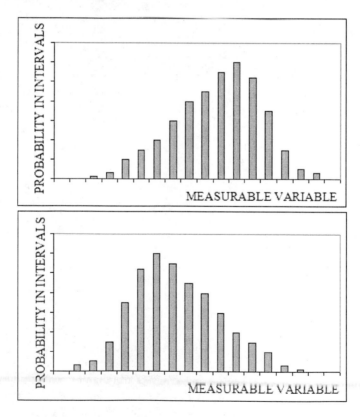

**Fig. 3.6.** The examples of diagonal distributions: right- and left-handed

The example of the compliance analysis of the age distribution in the group of men and women with the SAS packet help is introduced in the workbook.

## THE FINAL REMARK

The statistical tests worked out by many authors and for many purposes are designed for analysing the sample and the features that describe those groups that represent the normal distribution and separately for those that do not represent such distribution. From the statistical procedures point of view, this differentiation is very important. The further procedure way in the statistical analysis depends upon the decision stating the accordance of empirical distribution with the theoretical (normal) one.

## Exercises

1. For the data, that you presented in the previous exercise as a histogram (empirical distribution), perform (using the tools available in Excel) the calculation of the $\chi^2$ test values (as shown in exercise part).
2. Consider the distribution chart shape for the left-handed distribution.
3. Using the tables at the end of the handbook (Supplement Tables), read the critical value of $\chi^2$ test, after the previous calculation of the freedom degrees and setting the significance level.
4. Make an objective decision with respect to $H_0$, by rejecting it (or stating that there are no reasons to reject $H_0$).
5. Interpret the decision.
6. Perform the same calculation for the second group of people (e.g. for those who did not survive the traffic accident).
7. Perform the Kolmogorov-Smirnov test, using the SAS program.
8. Compare the results obtained with your own calculations and those that you obtained by means of SAS packet.

# STEP 3 – exercise

# Checking the type of distribution

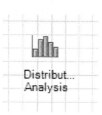

Distribut...
Analysis

We know all values that are needed to calculate the value of $\chi^2$ test to facilitate the objective evaluation of differences between the theoretical and empirical distribution. Before the value of $\chi^2$ test can be calculated, the limit condition for this test shall be satisfied. Namely, this test does not accept the frequency lower than 5 in each class. This is why the first class got incorporated to the second one and the last one to the before-last class. The $\chi^2$ test value can be calculated according to the formula given in Fig. 3.1. (formula bar).

| E2 | | ▼ | $f_x$ =((C2-D2)^2)/D2 | |
|---|---|---|---|---|
| A | B | C | D | E |
| 1 CLASSES | NUMBER | PR. OBS. | PR.THEOR. | ((PT-PO)^2)/PT |
| 2 <27] | 12 | 0.1291 | 0.0936 | 0.013464209 |
| 3 (27;39] | 14 | 0.1505 | 0.1318 | |
| 4 (39;51] | 9 | 0.0967 | 0.1996 | |
| 5 (51;63] | 23 | 0.2473 | 0.2214 | |
| 6 (63,75] | 13 | 0.1398 | 0.1801 | |
| 7 (75;99] | 22 | 0.2365 | 0.1541 | |
| 8 TOTAL | 19 | 0.9999 | 0.9806 | |

**Fig. 3.1.** Operations facilitating the calculation of the components of the sum to get the overall value of $\chi^2$ test. The formula bar contains a formula to calculate the components

The extension of the formula and calculation of the sum of the components are shown in Fig. 3.1. The same operation (elimination of classes represented by lower than 5 elements) shall be performed (Fig. 3.3.).

| | A | B | C | D |
|---|---|---|---|---|
| 1 | CLASSES | FREQ. | EMPIR. PROB. | THEOR. PROBABIL. |
| 2 | (3;15] | 3 | 0.0322 | 0.0298 |
| 3 | (15;27] | 7 | 0.0753 | 0.0638 |
| 4 | (27;39] | 17 | 0.183 | 0.1318 |
| 5 | (39;51] | 10 | 0.1074 | 0.1996 |
| 6 | (51;63] | 20 | 0.215 | 0.2214 |
| 7 | (63;75] | 15 | 0.1613 | 0.18 |
| 8 | (75;87] | 19 | 0.2043 | 0.1073 |
| 9 | (87;99] | 2 | 0.0215 | 0.0468 |
| 10 | TOTAL | 93 | 1 | 0.9805 |

**Fig. 3.2.** Data needed to compare the theoretical and empirical distribution. There is also the value of the sums to get the overall value of the $\chi^2$ test statistic

The value of the $\chi^2$ test statistic requires multiplication of the sum by the number of components in the sample.

| | A | B | C | D | E |
|---|---|---|---|---|---|
| 1 | CLASSES | NUMBER | PROB. OBSERV. | PROB. THEORET. | ((PT-PO)^2)/PT |
| 2 | <27] | 12 | 0.1291 | 0.0936 | 0.013464209 |
| 3 | (27;39] | 14 | 0.1505 | 0.1318 | 0.002653187 |
| 4 | (39;51] | 9 | 0.0967 | 0.1996 | 0.053048146 |
| 5 | (51;63] | 23 | 0.2473 | 0.2214 | 0.003029855 |
| 6 | (63;75] | 13 | 0.1398 | 0.1801 | 0.009017712 |
| 7 | (75;99] | 22 | 0.2365 | 0.1541 | 0.04406074 |
| 8 | TOTAL | | 0.9999 | 0.9806 | 0.12527385 |

**Fig. 3.3.** Value of the $\chi^2$ test statistic. The formula bar contains a formula facilitating the computation of the value of the $\chi^2$ test statistic

The value of $\chi^2$ test may be calculated multiplying the sum (0.125) by the number of elements in the sample e.q. 93. The final result is 11.62. The critical value of $\chi^2$ test distribution for 5 degrees of freedom for significance = 5% is 11.070. As the calculated value is greater than the critical one for $\chi^2$ test, the null hypothesis should be rejected. It means that the distribution of ages among women with nephrolithiasis is not normal.

If we perform an identical analysis for men we obtain a table as shown in Fig. 3.4.

| | A | B | C | D | E |
|---|---|---|---|---|---|
| 1 | CLASSES | NUMBER | PROB. OBSERV. | PROB. THEORET. | ((PT-PO)^2)/PT |
| 2 | <24] | 13 | 0.079754601 | 0.0589 | 0.007383946 |
| 3 | (24;36] | 27 | 0.165644172 | 0.1449 | 0.002969777 |
| 4 | (36;48] | 55 | 0.337423313 | 0.2594 | 0.023468147 |
| 5 | (48;60] | 39 | 0.239263804 | 0.2767 | 0.00506494 |
| 6 | (60;72] | 21 | 0.128834356 | 0.1761 | 0.012686207 |
| 7 | (72;84] | 8 | 0.049079755 | 0.0836 | 0.014254155 |
| 8 | TOTAL | 163 | 1 | 0.9996 | 0.065827171 |

**Fig. 3.4.** Data needed to calculate the value of the $\chi^2$ test statistic. There is also the value of the $\chi^2$ test for this sample

The critical value of $\chi^2$ test distribution with 5 degrees of freedom for significance = 5% is 11.070. The calculated value for $\chi^2$ test is equal to 10.72. In this case we have no reason to reject the null hypothesis, which means that the probability distribution of ages among men is normal.

| F | $\chi^2$ CALCUL. | 11.642 |
|---|---|---|
| DF = 5 | $\chi^2$ CRIT. | 11.070 |
| | | |
| M | $\chi^2$ CALCUL. | 10.722 |
| DF = 5 | $\chi^2$ CRIT. | 11.070 |

**Fig. 3.5.** Final results of $\chi^2$ test including critical values in females and males

So far we finished our work in Excel. No we start the analysis in the SAS environment. After loading the data (using the Import Data option) we get a dialog box as shown below. The content of our database is displayed in the lower part of the screen.

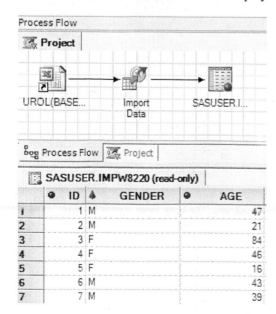

**Fig. 3.6.** Dialog box of the SAS program. In the upper part we can see the graphic representation of the consecutive steps: load of data (UROL(BASE...) using the Import Data option. If the data have been loaded correctly, the SAS database (SASUSER) is created. All references to the primary data are references to this icon. The lower portion of the drawing shows part of the database used in the calculation

A selection of options pertaining to analysis of the type of distribution (**Distribution Analysis ...**) is available on the main toolbar **Analyze** (Fig. 3.7.).

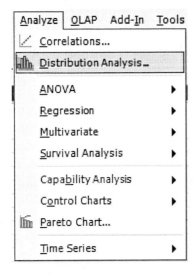

**Fig. 3.7.** After extending the Analyze option, we can further specify our selection, which is Distribution Analysis in this case

To perform distribution analysis, similar to all other calculations, we need to define the characteristics we want to analyze (Fig. 3.8.).

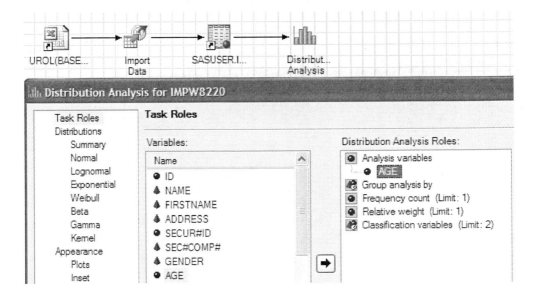

**Fig. 3.8.** Other options related to the previously selected procedure (test) are available via a dialog box where a first step is always to select variables to be analyzed. Here we analyze age and this characteristic is selected from the list of variables

Various distributions are available and we should select the expected distribution. In our case it is only normal distribution (presentation of other distributions is outside the scope of this book).

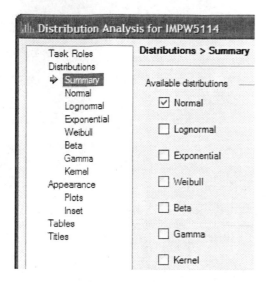

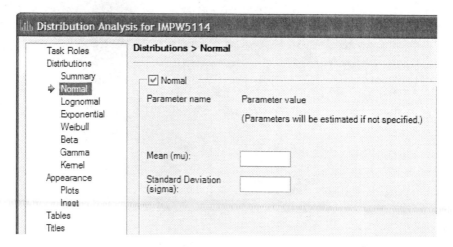

**Fig. 3.9.** We select the type of distribution we want to analyze. Here it is normal distribution

In this dialog box we selected the distribution we want to find. Other distributions are beyond the scope of this book.

It is not enough to define the type of distribution (Fig. 3.10.). We must specify further conditions in another dialog box.

**Fig. 3.10.** In this dialog box we enter two parameters of the normal distribution (the mean and standard deviation). As we may see these values may be calculated automatically by the program

In the new dialog box you select a graphic presentation of the distribution (Fig. 3.11.).

**Distribution Analysis for IMPW5114**

Task Roles
Distributions
    Summary
    Normal
    Lognormal
    Exponential
    Weibull
    Beta
    Gamma
    Kernel
Appearance
  ⇨ Plots
    Inset
Tables
Titles

**Appearance > Plots**

Note: Insets are valid on histogram, probability and quantile-quantile plots only.

☑ Histogram Plot

☐ Probability Plot

☐ Quantiles plot

☐ Box plot

☑ Stem and leaf text plot

**Fig. 3.11.** In the new dialog box you select a graphic presentation of the distribution. Here two graphic presentations have been selected

Other dialog boxes are available after clicking on the **Run** option in the lower part of the screen.

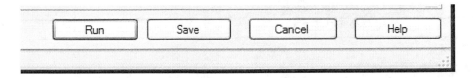

| Run | Save | Cancel | Help |

**Fig. 3.12.** Bar in the lower part of the screen. After clicking the Run option you go to another page. If this option is inactive (dull) it means an error when entering the data or no data entered to perform this task

The dialog box and options presented above facilitate the performance of distribution analysis. We plan to perform this analysis separately for men and women.
In order to obtain these two groups we have to execute filter procedure.
Filter procedure is available via the **Data** option.

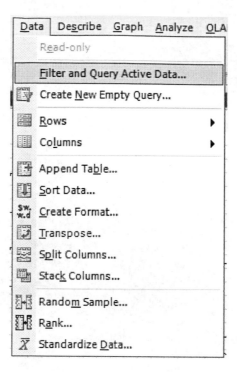

**Fig. 3.13.** Filter allows extracting only part of data records to analyze. Query allows you to specify the criteria for blocking out data

In this dialog box you may specify the criteria for the records. A full set of features is listed in the left panel. Click on the field's name, hold down the button, drag and drop the object in the right panel.

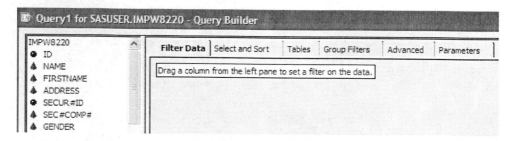

**Fig. 3.14.** A list of variables is displayed in the dialog box. Selecting the variable means that this feature serves as a criterion for blocking out data

You have defined the feature that serves as the criteria for the records. Now you have to specify filter conditions. Gender is coded as F and M. The program understands these symbols as text. If you want to block out records with the symbol "F", select =*,**LIKE, character pattern maching**. In this example the identified code sounds like K. The program must know that it is a letter symbol and thus the letter K should be given in parentheses.

If you use numeric data, select =,**equals** and provide its value.

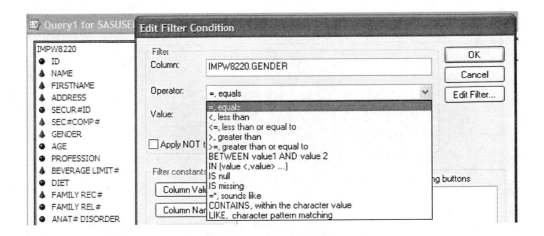

**Fig. 3.15.** GENDER has been selected (upper part of the right window). We select sounds like (gender is entered as letters F and M)

The correctly defined filter condition is shown below. The **Apply NOT to filter** box is also important. If you tick this box, the final database will contain records with gender code M.

| Edit Filter Condition | | |
|---|---|---|
| **Filter**<br>Column: IMPW8220.GENDER | | OK |
| | | Cancel |
| Operator: LIKE, character pattern matching | | Edit Filter... |
| Value: 'F| | | |
| ☐ Apply NOT to filter | | |

**Fig. 3.16.** Specifying the criteria for blocking out data, here it is – GENDER – which if sounds like "F" will be eliminated from further analysis

The end of the filtering operation is shown below. Once the query is entered, it may be executed by clicking on the **RUN** button.

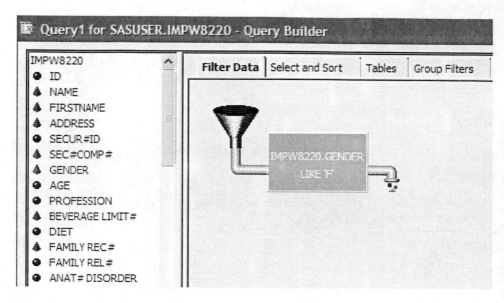

**Fig. 3.17.** Selecting the RUN button will create a sub-base of women

Below there are the results of a non-parametric test stating whether there are any differences or similarities between two samples with respect to age. Remember the null hypothesis which is "Both samples are derived from the same population". If the differences are found, it means that the females and males do not make up a homogenous population. Note that this test does not analyze any parameters (arithmetic mean, median etc.).

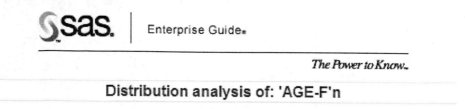

### Distribution analysis of: 'AGE-F'n

*The UNIVARIATE Procedure*
*Variable: AGE-F (AGE-F)*

The **Univariate procedure** is the appropriate procedure in SAS language.

| Basic Statistical Measures | | | |
|---|---|---|---|
| **Location** | | **Variability** | |
| **Mean** | 55.01075 | **Std Deviation** | 21.24418 |
| **Median** | 56.00000 | **Variance** | 451.31510 |
| **Mode** | 54.00000 | **Range** | 88.00000 |
| | | **Interquartile Range** | 36.00000 |

**Fig. 3.18.** The heading of the procedure that tests the conformity of the empirical distribution to the normal distribution and a table of results (descriptive analysis of the sub-base created after elimination of males from the database)

Irrespective of the test conditions, the mean and standard deviation have been calculated. These values may be obtained for any set of data. In a situation in which the distribution of a given feature is normal, the mean and standard deviation are the parameters of the normal distribution. In other situations, these values may also be obtained, but they are not the parameters of any distribution.

| Basic Confidence Limits Assuming Normality | | | |
|---|---|---|---|
| **Parameter** | **Estimate** | **95% Confidence Limits** | |
| **Mean** | 55.01075 | 50.63557 | 59.38594 |
| **Std Deviation** | 21.24418 | 18.56828 | 24.82831 |
| **Variance** | 451.31510 | 344.78116 | 616.44484 |

**Fig. 3.19.** Calculation of confidence intervals for the mean and standard deviation, and variance

The table above provides the confidence interval for the mean and standard deviation.

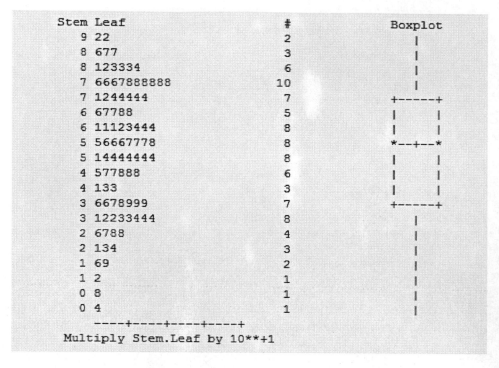

```
Stem Leaf                              #          Boxplot
   9 22                                2             |
   8 677                               3             |
   8 123334                            6             |
   7 6667888888                       10             |
   7 1244444                           7          +------+
   6 67788                             5          |      |
   6 11123444                          8          |      |
   5 56667778                          8          *--+--*
   5 14444444                          8          |      |
   4 577888                            6          |      |
   4 133                               3          |      |
   3 6678999                           7          +------+
   3 12233444                          8             |
   2 6788                              4             |
   2 134                               3             |
   1 69                                2             |
   1 2                                 1             |
   0 8                                 1             |
   0 4                                 1             |
       ----+----+----+----+
 Multiply Stem.Leaf by 10**+1
```

**Fig. 3.20.** Results showing the empirical distribution. Age of the females is given on the left side. The second column provides the number of subjects in a given class. A simplified distribution on the right side shows the location of the mean (+) and the range that contains 68% of the results. The + sign is in the middle of the box, which means that the distribution is skewed

The drawing above shows the distribution of age in a simplified form. How to interpret this drawing? The first (left) column provides the number of tens, whereas the space is followed by the values of units. Therefore, in our group there are subjects who are 12, 16 and 17 years old. The column in the middle of the panel provides the number of subjects in a given age group (classes divided according to tens of years).

Because of different numbers of subjects in the groups, the drawing resembles a tree with its top identifying the largest group of subjects.

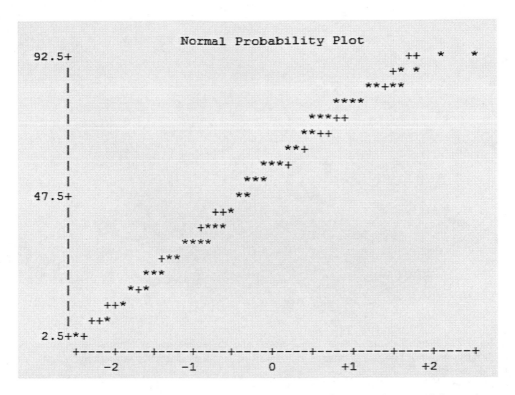

**Fig. 3.21.** Graphic presentation of the results. The vertical axis shows the age of the patients. The horizontal axis shows the normal order statistic means or medians

The drawing above displays the relations among the expected – conforming to the normal distribution – number of subjects. The data are plotted in such a way that the points should form a straight line, departures from that line indicate the differences form normality.

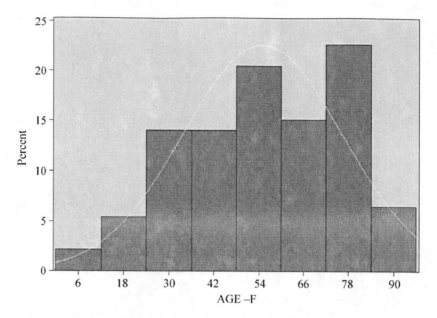

**Fig. 3.22.** Empirical distribution (histogram) and the superimposed normal distribution line (continuous line). The plot compares the theoretical and the empirical distribution

The bar chart above is a histogram showing how age is distributed in the group of female patients. Bars indicate the observed frequencies and the yellow line refers to the normal distribution. You may subjectively evaluate differences between the empirical, observed and the theoretical, expected distribution.

| Parameters for Normal Distribution | | |
|---|---|---|
| **Parameter** | **Symbol** | **Estimate** |
| **Mean** | Mu | 55.01075 |
| **Std Dev** | Sigma | 21.24418 |

**Fig. 3.23.** Another table with the arithmetic mean and standard deviation

The values for the normal distribution calculated for our dataset.

| Goodness-of-Fit Tests for Normal Distribution | | | | |
|---|---|---|---|---|
| Test | | Statistic | | p Value |
| Kolmogorov-Smirnov | D | 0.09387056 | Pr > D | 0.043 |
| Cramer-von Mises | W-Sq | 0.11842204 | Pr > W-Sq | 0.066 |
| Anderson-Darling | A-Sq | 0.77074896 | Pr > A-Sq | 0.045 |

**Fig. 3.24.** Results of statistical tests testing the goodness-of-fit of observed to expected distributions. The Kolmogorov-Smirnov goodness-of-fit test is discussed here. The p value is less than the chosen 5% significance level and therefore $H_0$ should be rejected. It means that the differences seen in Fig. 3.20. are statistically significant and consequently, the ages in female patients with nephrolithiasis are not normally distributed

Here you will find results of three independent tests showing close agreement between the empirical and theoretical distribution. The other two tests are not discussed in this reference book. The p value of the Kolmogorov-Smirnov test is less than 5%, which means that $H_0$ should be rejected. It means further that the ages of female patients in our population are not normally distributed.

| Quantiles for Normal Distribution | | |
|---|---|---|
| Quantile | | |
| Percent | Observed | Estimated |
| 1.0 | 4.00000 | 5.58940 |
| 5.0 | 19.00000 | 20.06719 |
| 10.0 | 27.00000 | 27.78524 |
| 25.0 | 38.00000 | 40.68177 |
| 50.0 | 56.00000 | 55.01075 |
| 75.0 | 74.00000 | 69.33973 |
| 90.0 | 82.00000 | 82.23626 |
| 95.0 | 86.00000 | 89.95432 |
| 99.0 | 92.00000 | 104.43210 |

**Fig. 3.25.** Table with empirical and estimated (expected) percentiles. Analyzing the differences, you may determine those intervals which are most discrepant from the estimated (expected) ones

Above you will find centiles (and quantiles). The larger the differences between "empirical" and "theoretical", the bigger the discrepancy between these two distributions.

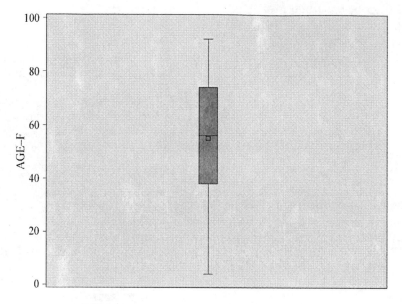

**Fig. 3.26.** Box-and-whisker plot. The vertical axis indicates values referring to age. The size of the box shows the $\bar{x} \pm s$, the horizontal line indicates the location of the arithmetic mean, and the small square the location of the median

The box-and-whisker plot (or simply boxplot) shows the location of the arithmetic mean (the horizontal line within the box), standard deviation (the size of the box), median (the small square in the box) and the interquartile range (whiskers).

A similar analysis is performed for male patients.

### Distribution analysis of: 'AGE-M'n

*The UNIVARIATE Procedure*
*Variable: AGE-M (AGE-M)*

| Basic Statistical Measures | | | |
|---|---|---|---|
| Location | | Variability | |
| Mean | 45.91411 | Std Deviation | 15.90419 |
| Median | 46.00000 | Variance | 252.94319 |
| Mode | 43.00000 | Range | 85.00000 |
| | | Interquartile Range | 19.00000 |

**Fig. 3.27.** Parameters referring to measures of location (mean, median and mode) and measures of spread (standard deviation, variance, range) in male patients

Descriptive analysis of age in male patients.

| Basic Confidence Limits Assuming Normality | | | |
|---|---|---|---|
| Parameter | Estimate | 95% Confidence Limits | |
| Mean | 45.91411 | 43.45418 | 48.37404 |
| Std Deviation | 15.90419 | 14.34486 | 17.84686 |
| Variance | 252.94319 | 205.77515 | 318.51035 |

**Fig. 3.28.** Confidence intervals for the mean, standard deviation and variance of age in male patients

Confidence intervals for the parameters of the normal distribution (see table above).

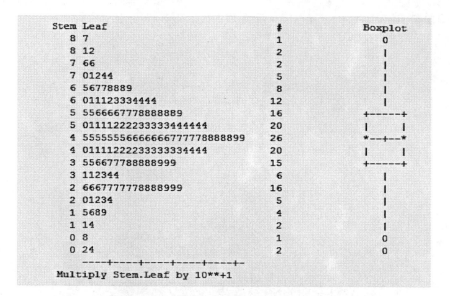

```
Stem Leaf                              #              Boxplot
  8 7                                  1                 0
  8 12                                 2                 |
  7 66                                 2                 |
  7 01244                              5                 |
  6 56778889                           8                 |
  6 011123334444                      12                 |
  5 5566667778888889                  16              +-----+
  5 01111222233333444444              20              |     |
  4 55555556666666777778888899        26              *--+--*
  4 01111222233333334444              20              |     |
  3 556677788888999                   15              +-----+
  3 112344                             6                 |
  2 6667777778888999                  16                 |
  2 01234                             5                  |
  1 5689                               4                 |
  1 14                                 2                 |
  0 8                                  1                 0
  0 24                                 2                 0
      ----+----+----+----+----+-
Multiply Stem.Leaf by 10**+1
```

**Fig. 3.29.** Distribution of ages in male patients. The interpretation is similar to that in Fig. 3.18.

The stem-and-leaf display represents a more complex distribution in the individual age groups in the female population.

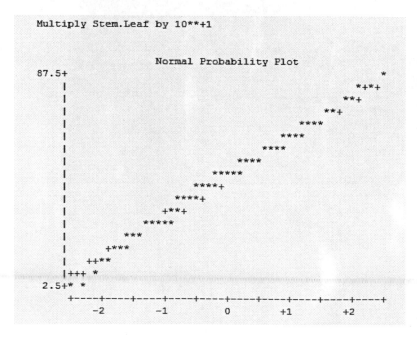

**Fig. 3.30.** Graphic display of age in the male population. The description is the same as in Fig. 3.19.

Discrepancies from the expected normal distribution (the + signs indicate that in a given age group there are more subjects than expected for the normal distribution).

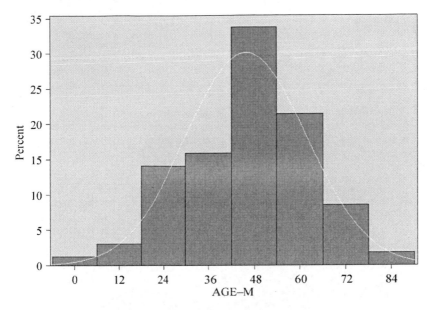

**Fig. 3.31.** Empirical distribution (blue histogram) and the superimposed normal distribution line (yellow) in the male population

The histogram above shows how age is distributed in the group of male patients. The height of the bars represents the number of patients in a given age group. The yellow line shows the theoretical relationship conforming to the normal distribution.

| Parameters for Normal Distribution | | |
|---|---|---|
| Parameter | Symbol | Estimate |
| Mean | Mu | 45.91411 |
| Std Dev | Sigma | 15.90419 |

**Fig. 3.32.** Parameters for normal distribution (Greek symbols mu, sigma)

The table provides the parameters for normal distribution that served as basis for drawing the yellow line of the theoretical distribution.

| Goodness-of-Fit Tests for Normal Distribution | | | | |
|---|---|---|---|---|
| Test | | Statistic | p Value | |
| Kolmogorov-Smirnov | D | 0.05964914 | Pr > D | >0.150 |
| Cramer-von Mises | W-Sq | 0.07029087 | Pr > W-Sq | >0.250 |
| Anderson-Darling | A-Sq | 0.37507206 | Pr > A-Sq | >0.250 |

**Fig. 3.33.** Results of goodness-of-fit tests for normal distribution. The Kolmogorov-Smirnov goodness-of-fit test is discussed here. The p value indicates that $H_0$ should be rejected. It means that there is a Gaussian function describing the empirical distribution (for the chosen acceptance of error)

Here you will find results of tests showing differences between the empirical and theoretical (normal) distribution. The Kolmogorov-Smirnov goodness-of-fit test is discussed here. This time the p value is more than 5%, meaning that there is no reason to reject $H_0$ which says that there is no difference between the theoretical normal) and empirical distribution.

| Quantiles for Normal Distribution | | |
|---|---|---|
| | Quantile | |
| Percent | Observed | Estimated |
| 1.0 | 4.00000 | 8.91544 |
| 5.0 | 19.00000 | 19.75405 |
| 10.0 | 26.00000 | 25.53207 |
| 25.0 | 37.00000 | 35.18690 |
| 50.0 | 46.00000 | 45.91411 |
| 75.0 | 56.00000 | 56.64132 |
| 90.0 | 66.00000 | 66.29615 |
| 95.0 | 71.00000 | 72.07417 |
| 99.0 | 82.00000 | 82.91278 |

**Fig. 3.34.** Quantiles of age distribution in the population of male patients

The table above provides values of the empirical and theoretical quantiles. In this case the differences between these values are much smaller than in the female population. It means that all age groups are represented as expected.

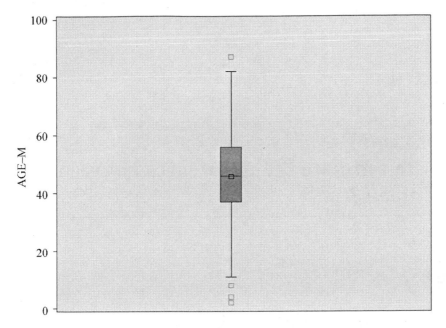

**Fig. 3.35.** Distribution of age in the male population (small squares outside the vertical line identify outliers)

This box-and-whisker plot slightly differs from the plot in the population of women. The blue small squares above and below the box are called outliers. There are various criteria for evaluating the outliers. Here we accept the interpretation of the SAS program.

In conclusion, we may state that the men's age – patients with nephrolithiasis – are normally distributed. The distribution of female ages is other than normal. This situation gives rise to a question: why the distribution of ages in the group of women with nephrolithiasis is other than normal and different than that in the group of men. The answer will be given in next chapters where statistical analysis is continued.

# STEP 4

## T-test and F-test
## How to estimate the differences between groups of patients?

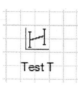

Test T

> **Do the patients, in whom the urinary tract infection was found, differ with their bodily temperature from those, in whom the bacteria were not found?**
>
> **Is the bodily temperature really different for the group with the haematuria found in relation to the group without haematuria?**

Both questions can be objectively answered by using the statistical tests, called: F-test (Snedecor's test) and Student's t-test (sometimes called T-test).[21]

The Gauss function, as well as the normal distribution are characterized by the fact that, apart from the dependence from the measured value $X$, the shape of the chart depends also on two parameters: the arithmetic mean and the standard deviation.

---

[21] The Author of a statistical test is entitled to name it. Sometimes that arbitrary freedom causes the emergence of unfamiliar and unintelligible test names.

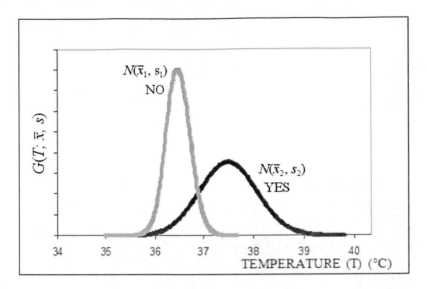

**Fig. 4.1.** The bodily temperature distribution of the patients (both men and women). The two groups differentiated in the illustration are the people, in urine of whom the bacteria were found (YES) and those, where bacteria were not found (NO)

Before we proceed to the comparative analysis of the two presented patients' groups, we shall refer to a simple example that was made by means of a suitable compilation of the example presented in Fig. 4.1 in order to explain a certain phenomenon.

Let us imagine that we are comparing two groups, in which the distribution of a given feature assumes the form like the one presented in Fig. 4.2.A, and another example, that is represented in Fig. 4.2.B as we can see, the values of arithmetic means for the sample AI and for the sample BI are comparable. The same can be told about the mean values AII and BII. Can we expect that the evaluation of differences between the two mean values AI and AII as well as between BI and BII at the same difference between them will be the same? A careful Reader is likely to notice that in the example A the two charts are completely separated. There is no such measurement in those groups, of which we could not say which group it belongs to. It is different in the example B. Here the charts overlap in a certain area. There are results from that overlapping area, whose ascribing to group I or II is a problem.

The whole consideration is aimed at suggesting that an analysis of the differences between the distributions and between the mean values are combined with each other. It is likely to be no wonder for the Reader, that the test evaluating the differences between the mean values will be preceded by the comparative analysis of dispersions, and that the values of standard deviation (variance) will appear also in the mathematical definition of the arithmetic mean values comparison criterion, because, as it is visible in the Fig. 4.2.A and Fig. 4.2.B, the dispersion value in the comparable groups has an essential meaning for the evaluation of the differences between the mean values in those groups.

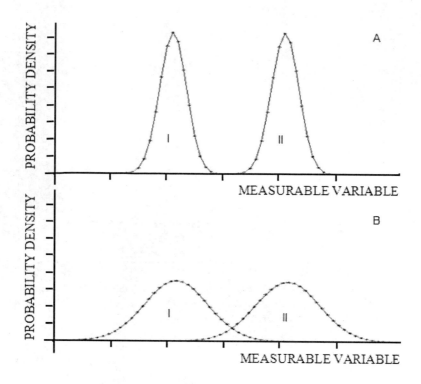

**Fig. 4.2.** The setting of two groups I and II in the cases of low standard deviation value (A) and high standard deviation value (B)

Coming back to our example of the patients' bodily temperature distribution in two groups distinctive for the bacteriuria, we should examine, the differences between this parameter in those two groups. The charts shown in Fig. 4.1. represent the feature distributions (THE SAME variable – one must not compare the distributions of different variables – and the common $X$-axis is a frequent students' error) in two groups. In both of them the presence of normal distribution for the bodily temperature feature has already been found (applying the goodness-of-fit test).

As it can be seen, the locations of the mean are different and the dispersion values also differ. The question is, if the values of differences are relevant or if they can be ignored. Such comparisons make sense only after the prior finding that there are possibilities of treating the empirical distribution as the normal distribution. In other words, in both cases we had to find out earlier that there is normal distribution, which represents our empirical distribution (the $\chi^2$ or Kolmogorov-Smirnov test). If the distribution is different than normal, though, we cannot test the parameters of the normal distribution (if the analysed feature does not represent such a distribution).

E.g. we cannot answer a question about the mean values differences and the age distribution in the male patients in proportion to female patients, as we have already stated that the age distribution in women is different than the normal one. We shall answer the question concerning the differences between the men's and the women's age in the further part of the handbook, using another test.

Because, as it has already been stated, **both distributions shown in Fig. 4.1. were estimated as normal distributions** (we do not present this procedure as we assume that each reader knows how to perform such a procedure). The condition of normal distribution in comparable groups shall be satisfied. We can treat both the arithmetic mean and the standard deviation (variance) as the parameters of the normal distribution. The statistical procedure provides first the distribution value comparative analysis and then the mean values comparison.

There is an important question concerning the bacteriuria in the patient (the urinary tract infection during the nephrolithiasis fit – the stone moves and hurts the organ's walls, which threatens the further infection of the blood circulation system and a basic danger to the patient's life and health). We shall check if the bodily temperature of the patients with bacteriuria is really higher in relation to those patients, in whom the bacteria in urine were not found.[22]

We shall refer to the familiar scheme of testing the statistical hypotheses procedure. According to what has been told above, the first to be compared are the variance values with the people with the positive bacteriuria analysis result and those, in whom no bacteriuria was found.

In case of comparing the variances (F-test) that represent two groups, that procedure assumes the following form:

---

[22] The arithmetic mean value can be calculated for any set of numbers. E.g. the mean value of two measurements of the given physiological fluid component concentration informs us, that two levels of that component concentration most probably oscillate around that value. That value differs in its interpretation in relation to the values of the mean calculated for the measurement results set, with which the Gaussian distribution presence was found. The arithmetic mean acts as a parameter in the expression for the Gaussian function. The Gaussian function depends on the $x$ variable (the value of our analyzed feature). Its shape is influenced by the parameter, which is the arithmetic mean. The illustration below presents the influence. The distribution that follows the Gauss function pattern is just situated on the number axis in the other area. A similar role of the parameter is performed by the standard deviation, whose value influences the Gaussian function form in the way presented in Fig. 4.1. That parameter (standard deviation) influences the bell curve width, which, of course, illustrates other distributions of the analyzed feature values. Comparing the two groups (and precisely – two distributions or two parameter sets of those distributions), we refer to the so-called parametric tests. In the light of the explanation presented above, that specification becomes obvious. Its obvious consequence, as one could infer, is also the presence of nonparametric tests in the statistical analysis (which will be discussed in the further part of the course).

1.  $H_0$ – there are no differences between the variances in two comparable groups.
    $H_1$ – there is a difference between the variances in two comparable groups.

2.  The objectiveness parameters:
    A – The number of degrees of freedom – the test is an exception among the statistical tests, and it expresses the freedom degrees number with two numbers. The number of freedom degrees is calculated separately for each group. And so, in the discussed text, the number of freedom degrees is calculated in the following way:

    $$df_1 = n_1 - 1 \qquad\qquad \text{(eq. 4.1.)}$$

    $$df_2 = n_2 - 1 \qquad\qquad \text{(eq. 4.2.)}$$

    B – The suggested significance level is 5%.

3.  The statistics value (the evaluation criterion):

    $$F = \frac{s_1^2}{s_2^2} \quad \text{if } s_1^2 > s_2^2, \qquad\qquad \text{(eq. 4.3.)}$$

    where $s_1^2$ – variance in group 1;

    $$F = \frac{s_2^2}{s_1^2} \quad \text{if } s_2^2 > s_1^2, \qquad\qquad \text{(eq. 4.4.)}$$

    where $s_2^2$ – variance in group 2.

4.  The critical value is read from the tables (the computer programme refers to the appropriate data stored in its memory).

    The critical value $F_{cr}(df_1, df_2, \alpha)$ – the specified critical area.

5.  We are making the final decision:

    $F_{cr}(df_1, df_2, \alpha) < F_{calc}$ – $H_0$ is rejected;

    $F_{cr}(df_1, df_2, \alpha) > F_{calc}$ – There is no reason to reject $H_0$.

6.  The final results interpretation.

The way of performing those calculations using the SAS program was shown in the workbook part.

We have found that the temperature distributions in the compared groups are different. There can be an interesting question why it happens so. Analysing the causes of such a state of affairs would require a further study (most probably biochemical). It may prove, though, that our further analysis will give an answer to this question. In the discussed case, the explanation seems simple, in case of bacteria presence the processes that mobilize the immunological system usually take place. There can be a rise in bodily temperature then, but there is no certainty in this respect. The rise in temperature can be considerable or not, depending on the bacteria strain and so-called general immunological resistance of the patient. Those patients in whom no bacteria were found have no reason for the rise in their bodily temperature, hence the higher uniformity (regarding the aspect of the bodily temperature feature) of this group of people.[23]

Using the statistical terminology we found that the variances in both groups were not uniform.

Regardless the F-test result, we can begin conducting the test that compares the arithmetic mean values (there are two versions of the test that compares the arithmetic mean values, with regard to the dependence on the relations between the variances). The test is called T-test (also called Student's t-test).

Referring again to the familiar procedure of testing the statistical hypotheses, we can specify the further stages of the test (test T) finding the significance (or the lack of significance) of the differences between the arithmetic mean values (the second parameter of the Gaussian function), that express the patient's bodily temperature in our example.

1. $H_0$ – there are no differences between the mean values in two compared groups.
   $H_1$ – there are differences between the mean values in two compared groups.

2. The objectiveness conditions:
   A – the number of degrees of freedom

$$df = n_1 + n_2 - 2; \qquad \text{(eq. 4.5.)}$$

   B – the significance level $\alpha = 5\%$.

3. The statistics value (the evaluation criterion): $H_0$
   T-test for the homogenous variances (the way of calculating the statistics values)

$$t = \frac{\overline{x}_1 - \overline{x}_2}{\sqrt{\dfrac{(n_1 - 1)s_1^2 + (n_2 - 1)}{n_1 + n_2 - 2}\left(\dfrac{1}{n_1} + \dfrac{1}{n_2}\right)}}, \qquad s_1^2, s_2^2 \; - \; \text{variances} \qquad \text{(eq. 4.6.)}$$

   T-test for the heterogeneous variances (the way of calculating the statistics values)

---

[23] It is obvious, that a patient can have a rise in the bodily temperature also for other reasons, but they are individual and do not influence the outlook of the whole, pretty numerous group of people.

$$u = \frac{\bar{x}_1 - \bar{x}_2}{\sqrt{\dfrac{s_1^2}{n_1} + \dfrac{s_2^2}{n_2}}}, \qquad s_1^2, \; s_2^2 \; - \; \text{variances} \qquad \text{(eq. 4.7.)}[24]$$

4. The critical value for the calculated values of degrees of freedom and the assumed significance level (found in the tables) $t_{cr}(\mu, \alpha)$.

5. The final decision:

$t_{cr}(\mu, \alpha) > T_{calc}$ – there are no grounds to reject $H_0$.

$t_{cr}(\mu, \alpha) < T_{calc}$ – $H_0$ is rejected.

6. Interpretation of final results.

An example of such an analysis was shown in the workbook part. The decision is: There is a statistically significant difference between average temperatures in the group of people with and without bacteriuria found.

The medical interpretation of the result obtained is simple. If the patient's bodily temperature is increased, the fact of urinary tract infection has to be taken into account. (the test result does not indicate with certainty that it really is so).

**However personally would we interpret Fig. 4.1., in relation to the arithmetic mean values and the distribution relation, an objective evaluation (by means of the tool, which is the statistical test) expresses the significant difference between the arithmetic mean values and the dispersion values (variances) of the patient's bodily temperature and without the bacteriuria found in the nephrolithiasis patient.**

Another question that we asked in the title of this chapter concerned the differences of the patient's bodily temperature when comparing the two groups – haematuria found, haematuria not found.

In the sample calculation (presented in the workbook part) we obtained the result: there are no grounds to reject $H_0$. It signifies that the temperature does not differentiate the patients' group from the aspect of haematuria.
There is no reason to link the presence of blood corpuscles in urine with any infectious process and there are no mechanisms that would explain the bodily temperature rise in case of the blood corpuscles' presence in urine. The processes responsible for their presence do not have (in their decisive majority) the character of infection.

---

[24] When presenting the above formulae, a certain simplification was introduced, which did not have much influence upon the practical procedure use.

To sum up, the increased bodily temperature may suggest the urinary tract infection, but does not suggest anything with respect to haematuria diagnosis.

We have referred several times to the critical values tables. What do the values in the tables signify and why does so much depend on them with respect to $H_0$?
We have frequently talked about the probability distributions and their characteristics. If, instead of the feature measured by the clinicians by its value whose distribution we are studying, it is the statistics value of any test, it will prove that certain values appear very often, and the other ones less frequently.

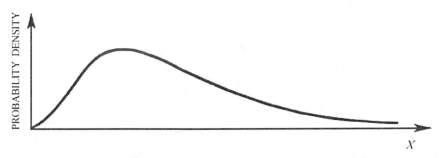

**Fig. 4.3.a.** A sample left-diagonal distribution for the values of the hypothetical X-test statistics (actually the curve represents the $\chi^2$ test distribution)

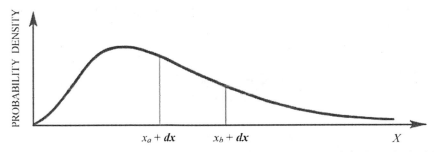

**Fig. 4.3.b.** A sample left-diagonal distribution for the statistics values of the hypothetical X-test. Equal rights are provided for all the distributions. Here, reading the probability values for the chosen values $x_a$ and $x_b$ was shown. The explanation of dX was given in STEP 2

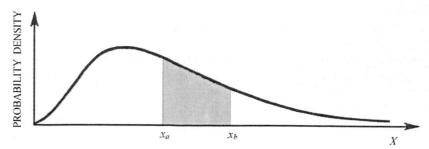

**Fig. 4.3.c.** A sample left-diagonal distribution for the statistics values of a hypothetical X-test. Equal rights are provided for all the distributions. Here, reading the values of range probability limited with the selected values $x_a$ and $x_b$ is presented. The grey area represents the sum of probability values (integral) for the selected range

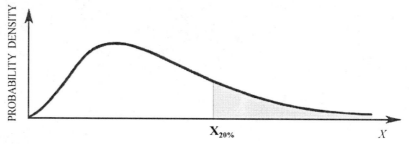

**Fig. 4.3.d.** A sample left-diagonal distribution for the statistics values of the hypothetical X-test. Equal rights are provided for all the distributions. Here, reading the values of range probability for the area comprising the highest values was shown. The selected area cuts off the highest values, whose probability of meeting equals 20%. The grey area represents the sum of probability values (integral) for the selected range

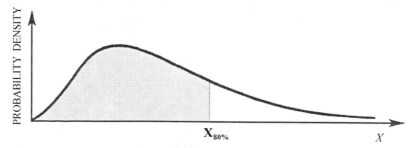

**Fig. 4.3.e.** A sample left-diagonal distribution for the statistics values of the hypothetical X-test. Equal rights are provided for all the distributions. of range probability for the area comprising the low values was shown. The grey area represents the sum of probability values (integral) for the selected range[25]

---

[25] A remark for the inquisitive ones: The illustrations present the probability distribution for the $\chi^2$ test values. As it can be seen, the distribution is conspicuously asymmetrical. The grey marked area in the lower illustration cuts on the $X$-axis the value, for which only five percent of

Fig. 4.2. a, b, c, d, e show the probability distribution of meeting the appropriate values of the test statistics (the $X$-axis marks the $\chi^2$ test values).

The statistical test Author is obliged to elaborate those distributions. We do not inquire into those procedures very deeply, as a mathematical training would be required, which reaches beyond the thematic scope of this handbook.

The majority of information (apart from the diagonality) concerning the probability distribution expressed with the Gauss function is also valid in relation to the $\chi^2$ test statistics values distribution.

And so, respectively, from the first illustration we learn that the distribution is diagonal (left-diagonal).

The probability values of obtaining a given $\chi^2$ value can be read as the point probability values.

The probability of appearance of the $\chi^2$ statistics value that belongs to the specific number range is expressed with the sum of the probability values for all the numbers from the marked range (it is represented graphically by the grey area).

If we are interested in very high values, which is to say the values expressing the highest possible differences between the variance values (expressed with the quotient), the value of the range probability should be calculated. If we are interested in a specific centile (e.g. 5%), the area has to be cut off that constitutes 5% of the whole surface under the curve. If we are interested in the range of $\chi^2$ values, that appear with the highest probabilities (e.g. 95%), the area of the surface marked in the next illustration should be calculated.

The last two pictures (Fig. 4.3.d and 4.3.e) are important for the further analysis and understanding the notion of so-called *critical area*.

We assumed that the analysis is done on the significance level of 5%. For such a condition from the penultimate chart we can read on the $X$-axis the value, which cuts 5% of all the results of high values. In that way we have found the critical value for the given significance level. If our value is calculated below the critical value defined in that way, it signifies that our result belongs to the group of results that constitute 95% of all the possible values of this test statistics. If we belong to such a large group, our result is nothing unusual. In that situation we state, that the difference is ignored. In other words, we did not find the reasons (premises) for finding the differences, and what follows is the final decision, which is the statement: "There are no grounds to reject the $H_0$ of this test".

If our calculated value is higher than the liminal value that cuts off 5% of results (the high values), it signifies that it is our result that belongs to those so rarely appearing high values. If we cut off the critical value just for that significance level it signifies, that we have exceeded the critical point and that the difference is not ignored any longer, and it has to be admitted as statistically significant.

---

tests obtain the result higher than the marked value. That illustration is a graphic presentation of the way of reading the critical value of the compliance $\chi^2$ test for the significance value level of 5%. Each calculated value higher than the abscissa signifies that our result is included in the set of those very rare values, and under those circumstances our difference is statistically insignificant.

Discussing the critical value, one more notion remains, the so-called **one- and two--sided test**.

In the example above we have discussed a situation, when the differences between the variance values where really considerable. A discussion of really negligible differences would miss a deeper sensibility. Thus we specify the $\chi^2$ test as a one-sided one.

It is different in case when the difference is high for the fact that one value is substantially higher and in the situation when one of the values is substantially lower than the other one. We talk about the double-sided test then. Both situations are presented in Fig. 4.4. and Fig. 4.5., which present the probability distribution of meeting various values of test t statistics. Coming back to the formula, according to which the statistics value of test t is calculated one should notice, that the mean values close to each other (there are no statistically significant differences) cause the appearance of the statistics value close to zero. The substantially different values can be expressed with a high positive value of t test and a high (in the absolute scale) negative value expressing the differences If we specify the significance level as equal to 5%, in such a situation, it can be perceived as single-sided, so we are interested in the relation of our statistics value calculated for a given example against the area cutting off the highest positive results (the illustration below). There is another possibility, though, when these 5% of extreme results encompasses both the high results (a high positive value) and the results substantially different at ht e negative value of statistics for the test t. In such a situation, the 5% area encompasses both the high and low values area. It should be noted, that the whole critical area is to express 5% of the surface under the curve.

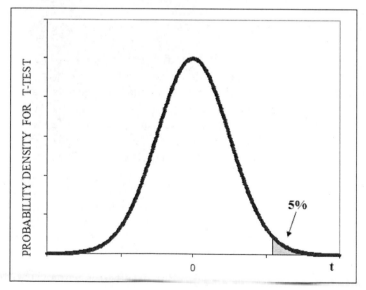

**Fig. 4.4.** The one-sided 5% critical area for the t-Student test[26]

---

[26] The distribution of the T-test values is very similar to normal distribution. This handbook does not get into details and is likely to admit neglecting the differences and operating with the normal distribution in order to explain the essence of the one- and two-sided test.

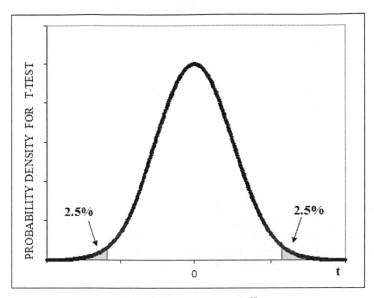

**Fig. 4.5.** The two-sided 5% critical area for the t-Student test[27]

It is important to specify at the beginning of the statistical analysis the significance level expressing the error value that we are ready to accept. In our example that significance level is 5%. As far as now, we have read the critical value corresponding to the chosen established significance level and according to the relation of the calculated and critical values, we made a decision concerning the $H_0$ purpose.

It can be done in another way, though, which is to say read the accumulated probability *"p"* for the statistics value calculated by us (the size of the area under the distribution curve for the $X$ value higher than our calculated value). If it proves, that the area is smaller than our assumed 5% it signifies, that our value is in the critical area (for the 5%), so in the same way we have proved, that our value belongs to those that appear rarely, and in that connection $H_0$ has to be rejected. Graphically, that situation (in relation to the probability distribution chart of the test F values occurrence) is presented in the illustration below:

---

[27] A remark for the inquisitive ones: The statistics values distribution for the t-Student test slightly differs from the normal distribution, yet the essence and the interpretation are common.

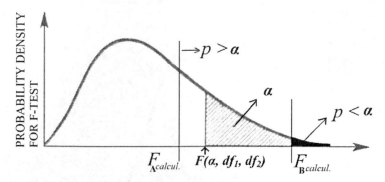

**Fig. 4.6.** The critical area of the F-Snedecor test (shaded area). Two different situations (A and B) are shown. One example with $F_{Acalcul.}$ where the F value is below $F(\alpha, df_1, df_2)$ and the second, when the $F_{Bcalcul.}$ is above the critical value $F(\alpha, df_1, df_2)$. It explains why in the first case there is no reason for rejection of $H_0$ and the second, why the $H_0$ shall be rejected

The advantage of using the *"p"* value in relation to referring to the critical value consists in the fact, that referring to the critical value imposes the qualitative meaning to the final decision on the $H_0$ rejection or not rejection. Using the *"p"* value has rather a quantitative character. The rejection of $H_0$ can follow a very slight majority of the calculated value in relation to the critical value (e.g. $F_{calc.} = 13.38$, $F_{crit.} = 11.07$). All the same, we shall reject $H_0$ when $F_{calc.} = 20.51$, and $F_{crit.} = 11.07$. Reading the *"p"* value for both sample values of the statistics $p1 = 2\%$ and $p2 = 0.001\%$ is a measure of the difference between the two values compared by us in this test.

We suggest analysing the above illustration that adequately represents the discussed problem.

There is one more essential remark concerning the statistical glossary of terms.
It has been written many times above that "$H_0$ is rejected". It signifies that we have proved that we found an example (our group of patients), in which the analysed parameter difference significance was demonstrated.
It has also been written that "There are no reason for the $H_0$ rejection". It does not signify that there are no differences between the mean values. It only signifies that with our data, we cannot prove the existence of the differences.

As we do not know the absolute truth, we agree to a certain defined error level, assumed by us. However, is a very low $\alpha$ always recommended? Assuming a very low $\alpha$ (e.g. 0.01%) causes, that although the statistics values difference (the value that specifies the estimation criterion) is very high (see the chart), we still declare that $H_0$ is not rejected. Minimizing the error of accepting the value of the statistics that indicates the differences presence, we enhance the probability of committing the contrary error. We are likely to neglect the difference (if $H_0$ tests the difference), that should already be treated as significant.

The table 4.1. explains the problem.

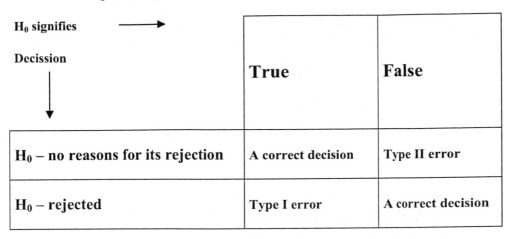

| H₀ signifies → Decission ↓ | True | False |
|---|---|---|
| **H₀ – no reasons for its rejection** | **A correct decision** | **Type II error** |
| **H₀ – rejected** | **Type I error** | **A correct decision** |

**Tab. 4.1.** The conditions for committing type I and type II error

The table implies that **type I error** (that is expressed exactly by means of the significance level $\alpha$) consists in the rejection of $H_0$ at the moment it is true. The lower value of the significance level we assume, the better we protect ourselves from the rejection of the correct $H_0$. Another possible error is the retention of the false $H_0$. This kind of error is specified as type II error. As a rule, when we diminish type I error, we automatically increase **type II error**. The type II error is strongly related to the power of the test.[28]

---

[28] The error type II is the probability of failing to reject the false null hypothesis and designed as $\beta$. The power of the test expressed as $1 - \beta$ measures the probability to that the false null hypothesis is rejected. The $\alpha$ is a single value assigned by the investigator in advance of performing the test. It is a measure of the acceptance risk to reject a true null hypothesis. In contrast to that, $\beta$ may be equal to one of many values. When false $II_0$ is failed to be rejected, the error type II is committed. The meaning of $\beta$ can be explained using the example shown in Fig. F1.A–D assuming that the $\bar{x}_1$, $\bar{x}_2$, or $\bar{x}_3$ represent the true unknown average values, the $\beta$ values can take different values respectively. The $\beta_1$ for example represents the level of the error type II for $\bar{x}_1$ to be true. Many numbers of possible values of the parameter under consideration (in our case the mean value) may be specified. This is why the power function (graphic presentation called power curve) is better assessment of the power of the test under consideration (Fig. F2.).

As it has already been said, the researcher looking for an answer to the specific question should state the significance level before beginning any procedures connected with collecting the data, as well as the experiment planning. The significance level

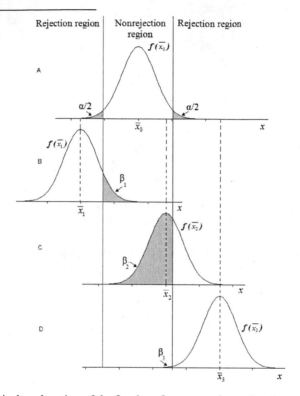

**Fig. F1.** The graphical explanation of the β values for mean value estimation

The $f(x)$ denotes the statistics test function oriented on the estimation of the mean values. The $\overline{x}_0$ is the value found on the basis of sample analysis. The values $\overline{x}_1$, $\overline{x}_2$ and $\overline{x}_3$ show the possible means (unknown) and the β values respectively.

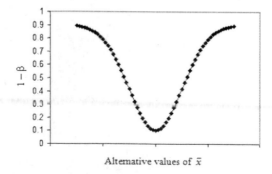

**Fig. F2.** The power curve for example shown in Fig. F1.

should be adequate with respect to the data accuracy and objectiveness (data collected at interviewing the patient, when the patient subjectively estimates his or her condition bear a high error and objectivity deficiency load, while e.g. laboratory analyses results, with the analyses performed with the adequate specialist equipment application bring objective information, void of accidental errors. Before starting a statistical analysis, the researcher should also realize consequences of the decisions he will make following the results obtained. If the results of the analysis made will only satisfy the researcher's curiosity, and the results are kept confidential, no consequences will be evoked, e.g. in relation to other people. However, if the research results are used for making the decisions upon which the others' fate will be corrected, the decision of assuming the adequate significance level should be considered very carefully. Moreover, if we prove the absence of detrimental side effects at the new medicine application, our decision will have meaningful consequences and may concern an enormous multitude of patients, for whom we take responsibility. How to adjust the significance level, then? Let us use an example. If we find that there are no differences between the side effects appearance in the control group (placebo applied) compared to the examined group (the new medicine applied), we want the effect to be the $H_0$ retention. We would rather reject the real $H_0$, even making type I error, than retain the false one. In such a situation, the significance level of 0.05 is correct. But if we are trying to prove that the medicine really influences the level of a specific component of the physiological fluids, the relevancy level should be the lowest possible, in order to be prevented from accepting the $H_0$ when it is false. In such a situation, the significance level equal 0.001 is adequate. If, in spite of so low significance level the $H_0$, is rejected, it signifies that the analysed and expected difference is really essential. It also signifies, that our result belongs to the set of results of a very low probabilities, which confirms its real credibility.

One should also remember that the fact of $H_0$ rejection signifies the explication of the significance differences between the comparable parameters. Stating no reason for $H_0$ rejection does not signify a declaration of the differences absence. It only signifies that we have not proved the presence of those differences by means of our sample.

**FINAL REMARKS**

To sum up, the obtained results of our analysis should be interpreted in the following way: In case of the bodily temperature rise in a patient, we can take into account the urinary tract infection. The connection between the bodily temperature and haematuria was not found.

# Exercises

1. Make a comparative analysis of the distribution and the arithmetic mean values of the feature that you consider essential from the point of view of traffic accidents casualties' analysis – remember of the prior statement of normal distribu-

tion in both groups. The division into groups (in order to find the normal distribution) can be obtained from SAS packet, using the „filter" (in the toolbar, after expanding the Data option). Then you will obtain the people who survived the accident, and separately those who died in it.

2. Make a series of F and T tests, asking other questions concerning e.g. the comparison of people, who needed further hospitalization in proportion to those, who did not need that type of treatment.

3. Compare the disability rate (expressed in %) between the people who suffered from burn in proportion to those in whom the burns were not found.

# STEP 4 – exercise

# F-test and T-test

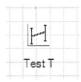

Test T

A test that compares variances and arithmetic means is accessible from the main menu in the following way:

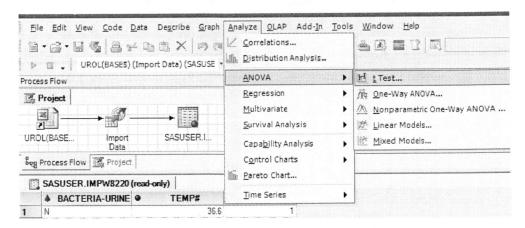

**Fig. 4.1.** Options dialog box showing how to perform Student's t-test. The Process Flow panel shows all standard steps for data loading

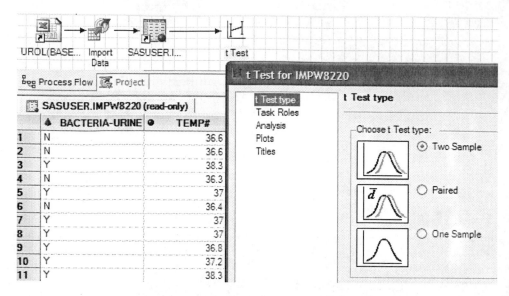

**Fig. 4.2.** In this dialog box we can choose the type of T-test: two sample test – to compare two independent patient groups – paired test to compare the results of clinical measurements in the same subjects obtained before and after treatment and one sample test – to compare the mean to specified value (which in particular may be zero). In this example you choose the two sample test. The left panel shows the stages of the calculation procedure relating to the test itself

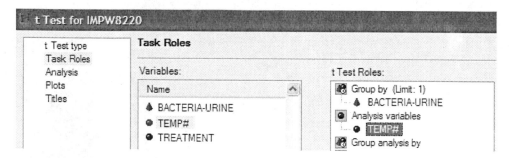

**Fig. 4.3.** Dialog box „Task Roles" to choose the features we want to analyze. Symbols in the right box describe the role of a given feature in a given test. The variable to be analyzed (here it is temperature) must be measurable (red ball) whereas the grouping variable may be qualitative or quantitative, provided that it assumes only two (not more) forms, because T-test is used to compare two groups

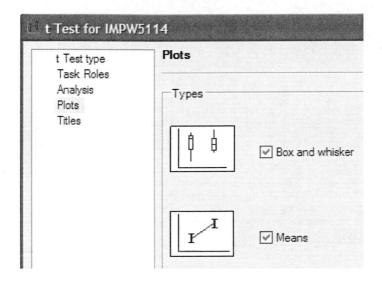

**Fig. 4.4.** In the Analysis box you specify the null hypothesis that there are no differences between the means (that's why 0) and define the confidence level (type I error)

**Fig. 4.5.** At this stage you specify the graphic display. In this example two available types have been ticked: a box and whisker plot and a means plot

| TEMP# | TEMP# | TEMP# | Variable |
|---|---|---|---|
| Diff·(1-2) | Y | N | BACTERIA URINE |
| 0 | 166 | 90 | N |
| -1.095 | 37.392 | 36.463 | Lower·CL Mean |
| -0.97 | 37.481 | 36.511 | Mean |
| -0.844 | 37.569 | 36.559 | Upper·CL Mean |
| 0.4465 | 0.5221 | 0.1989 | Lower·CL Std·Dev |
| 0.4853 | 0.5784 | 0.2281 | Std°Dev |
| 0.5315 | 0.6483 | 0.2673 | Upper·CL Std·Dev |
| 0.0635 | 0.0449 | 0.024 | Std°Err |
| 0 | 36 | 36 | Minimum |
| | 40 | 36.8 | Maximum |

Statistics

**Fig. 4.6.** The table summarizes temperatures measured in two groups with (Y) and without (N) bacteria in urine, the number of patients in each group, measures of location and variances with confidence intervals for the calculated parameters

| T-Tests | | | | | |
|---|---|---|---|---|---|
| Variable | Method | Variances | DF | t Value | Pr > \|t\| |
| TEMP# | Pooled | Equal | 254 | -15.66 | <.0001 |
| TEMP# | Satterthwaite | Unequal | 242 | -19.21 | <.0001 |

**Fig. 4.7.** The table summarizes T-test results (column 5). Degrees of freedom are given in column 4. Temperature is the variable we compare. As we said before the T-test has two versions depending on variances in the groups being compared. In this example both versions were applied. The upper line refers to equal variance and the lower line to unequal variance. You may decide which of these results is correct if you compare the variances as shown below

| Equality of Variances | | | | | |
|---|---|---|---|---|---|
| Variable | Method | Num DF | Den DF | F Value | Pr > F |
| TEMP# | Folded F | 165 | 89 | 6.43 | <.0001 |

**Fig. 4.8.** The table summarizes F-test results for equality of variances in the groups being compared providing degrees of freedom, F value and probability "p" which is very low. The final result of this test suggests rejecting $H_0$, which indicates that the variances are unequal. This result shows that in our example the result of t-test for unequal variances is correct (lower line). These tests prove that both variances and means are different in the two groups

| T-Tests | | | | | |
|---|---|---|---|---|---|
| Variable | Method | Variances | DF | t Value | Pr > \|t\| |
| TEMP# | Pooled | Equal | 254 | −15.26 | <.0001 |
| TEMP# | Satterthwaite | Unequal | 237 | −19.04 | <.0001 |

**Fig. 4.9.** Results of T-tests – in our example the lower line is correct due to the F-test result revealing the unequality of variances in two compared groups

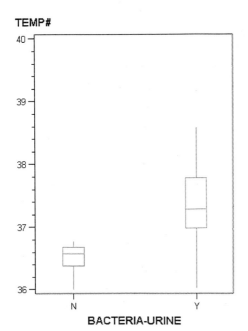

**Fig. 4.10.** A box and whisker plot (as selected in one of the previous dialog boxes) showing the location of the means (along the vertical axis) and values declared in the former step (selection of options for graphic presentation – in this case – 25% and 75% centyl) for the group with bacteria in urine – YES and without bacteria in urine – NO. The significant inequality of the means indicates that patients with bacteria in urine have higher mean temperatures

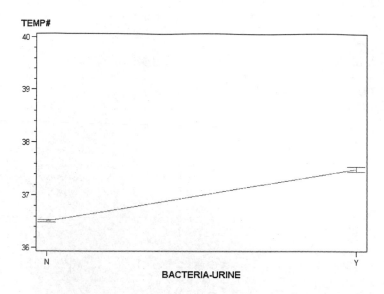

**Fig. 4.11.** Another graphic display of arithmetic means in the two groups with (Y) and without (N) bacteria in urine

| TEMP# | TEMP# | TEMP# | Variable | |
|---|---|---|---|---|
| Diff (1-2) | Y | N | BLOOD-URINE | |
| | 181 | 55 | N | |
| −0.057 | 37.027 | 37.08 | Lower CL Mean | |
| 0.1258 | 37.116 | 37.242 | Mean | |
| 0.3086 | 37.205 | 37.404 | Upper CL Mean | Statistics |
| 0.5527 | 0.5475 | 0.5037 | Lower CL Std Dev | |
| 0.6027 | 0.604 | 0.5984 | Std Dev | |
| 0.6627 | 0.6735 | 0.7371 | Upper CL Std Dev | |
| 0.0928 | 0.0449 | 0.0807 | Std Err | |
| | 0 6 | 36 3 | Minimum | |
| | 38.6 | 38.8 | Maximum | |

**Fig. 4.12.** The table shows the descriptive analysis of the temperature in two group of patients with (Y) and without (N) blood in urine

| T-Tests | | | | | |
|---|---|---|---|---|---|
| Variable | Method | Variances | DF | t Value | Pr > \|t\| |
| TEMP# | Pooled | Equal | 234 | 1.36 | 0.1765 |
| TEMP# | Satterthwaite | Unequal | 90 | 1.36 | 0.1765 |

**Fig. 4.13.** Results of T-tests comparing mean temperatures in patients with and without blood in urine. High "p" values suggest that there is no reason to say that the patients differ in mean body temperature

| Equality of Variances | | | | | |
|---|---|---|---|---|---|
| Variable | Method | Num DF | Den DF | F Value | Pr > F |
| TEMP# | Folded F | 180 | 54 | 1.02 | 0.9637 |

**Fig. 4.14.** The table summarizes F-test results showing no significant differences in variances of temperature between patients with and without blood in urine. The correct results of T-tests are given in the upper line of the previous table

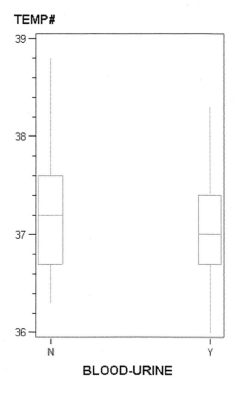

TEMP#

BLOOD-URINE

**Fig. 4.15.** The box and whisker plot presenting the result of the analysis of the patients' temperature in two groups of patients: with (Y) and without (N) blond in urine. Whiskers show the 25 and 75 centiles

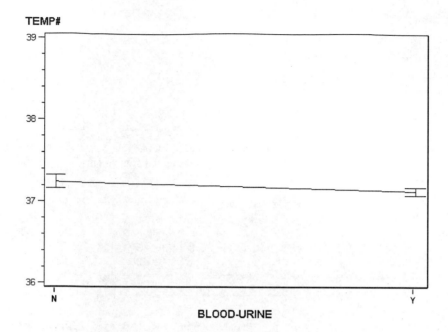

**Fig. 4.16.** The graphic presentation of the analysis of the patients' temperature in two groups: with (Y) and without (N) blood in the patients' urine. The horizontal line links the positions of the mean values and the brackets represents the interval of mean value ± standard deviation

# STEP 5

## ANOVA test
## How to compare more than two groups?

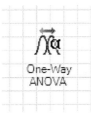

One-Way
ANOVA

> **Do the patients with different stone localization differ with the body temperature?**
>
> **Is the urine pH in patients with different chemical stone composition different?**

Very frequently in the analysis of a medical problem (as in our example) we conduct a comparison of a larger number of groups (not necessarily two). In such a situation, we refer to the ANOVA test (*ANalysis Of VAriance*).

In case of our analysis, we pose a question concerning the differences on the pH of patients urine, who we differentiate with respect to the chemical compounds.
The arrangement of the analysed data in the test described is shown in Fig. 5.1.

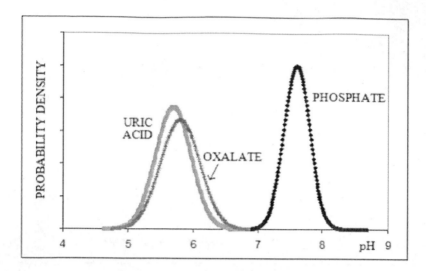

**Fig. 5.1.** Distributions of urine pH values in the groups differentiated for the stone composition

The testing procedure form is compliant with the already learned:

1. $H_0$ – there are no differences between the measurable feature mean values of the tested groups.
   $H_1$ – there are statistically significant differences between the measurable feature mean values of the comparable groups (at least two groups significantly differ from each other).

2. Objectivity conditions:
   A – the degrees of freedom number $df_1$, $df_2$ (the way of assigning is given in the table below),
   B – the significance level – we continue with the assumed $\alpha = 5\%$.

3. The value of statistics (the evaluation criterion) – a pretty complicated procedure (it requires calculating the values of $\bar{x}$ and $\bar{\bar{x}}$ ) – given in the table below.

$$\bar{x}_i = \frac{1}{n_i} \sum_{j=1}^{n_i} x_{ij} \quad \text{for} \quad i = 1, 2, ..., k \qquad \text{(eq. 5.1.)}$$

$$\bar{\bar{x}} = \frac{1}{n} \sum_{i=1}^{k} \sum_{j=1}^{n_i} x_{ij}, \quad \text{where} \quad n = \sum_{i=1}^{k} n_i \qquad \text{(eq. 5.2.)}$$

| Variability source | Sum of squares | Degrees of freedom | Variance | |
|---|---|---|---|---|
| Between populations (groups) | $\sum_{i=1}^{k}(\bar{x}_i - \bar{\bar{x}})^2 n_i$ | $K-1$ | $\hat{s}_1^2$ | $\hat{s}_{inter}^2$ |
| Within group (random component) | $\sum_{i=1}^{k}\sum_{j=1}^{n_i}(x_{ij} - \bar{x}_i)^2$ | $N-k$ | $\hat{s}_2^2$ | $\hat{s}_{intra}^2$ |

$$F = \frac{\hat{s}_1^2}{\hat{s}_2^2} \qquad\qquad F = \frac{\hat{s}_{inter}^2}{\hat{s}_{intra}^2}$$

(eq. 5.3.)

**4.** The critical value $F_{cr}(df_1, df_2, \alpha)$ – critical area.

**5.** The final decision.

$F_{calc.} < F_{cr}(\alpha, df_1, df_2)$     no reason to reject $H_0$

$F_{calc.} > F_{cr}(\alpha, df_1, dfr_2)$     $H_0$ rejected

**6.** Interpretation of final results.

Because we already know another method of showing the location of calculated statistics value with the *"p"* value,
The decisions made upon the calculated by the programme *"p"* value are the following:

**7.** The final decision:

**If the calculated "p" value < α significance level, $H_0$ is rejected.**

**If the calculated "p" value > α significance level, we state that there are no grounds for the $H_0$ rejection.**

The ANOVA test performed for the given example suggested the necessity to reject the $H_0$.
Rejecting $H_0$ signifies the presence of the differences between the mean values of the pH of urine in comparable groups (classified according to the chemical compound of the compound). It means that the presence of particular chemical compound influences the pH of urine.

Another example of applying the ANOVA test concerning the differences between the mean value of patients bodily temperature in the groups created with respect to the chemical composition of the stone. The calculation results revealed no significant differences between bodily temperature for groups generated according to their bodily temperature. It means, we cannot speculate about the chemical composition of the stone on the basis of known bodily temperature.

In our case it has been stated that there are no grounds for rejecting $H_0$. We can state then, that the rise in the bodily temperature for all the comparable groups created with respect to the crystalline deposit localization is comparable. In other words, it can be told that the localization of the stone has no specific connection with the human body temperature rise.[29]

As it can be seen, the mean value of the urine pH is differentiated with respect to the category of chemical compound that is accumulated in the urinary tract. It results from the chemical characteristics of the compounds that appear in the stones deposited in the urinary tract.

There are compounds, whose solubility diminishes with the acidity of the solution, other act in the contrary way. Hence, upon the urine pH, one can suppose what the main component of the stone is. The analysis of the stone chemical composition is rather expensive and complicated (highly specific equipment is needed). So, if a quick estimate of the kind of stone is needed, one can suppose, of course with a certain approximation, what the main component of the stone is, by interpreting the patient's urine pH value. The estimation of the stone composition is essential for therapy. The efficiency of new lithotripsy technology depends is strongly on the chemical compound deposited in urinary system.

---

[29] The above schedule of conducting the ANOVA test needs additional explanations.

The basis to make a comparison of the differences between the mean values is comparing the variance (which may appear strange, as we are comparing the mean values). Nevertheless, it proves quite justified. The idea consists in stating whether the distributions of the mean values (there are several of them, so their distribution can be estimated) against the global mean value (the mean value calculated for all the elements together, irrespectively of their affiliation to a specific group) is substantially different with respect to the variance distribution in particular groups. In other words, if the values distributions within the groups are comparable to the spread between the mean values, we can say that the groups do not differ between one another. If we find that the spread between the mean values is substantially higher in relation to the spreads within the groups, one could expect that the groups differ one from another from the point of view of the arithmetic mean values.

Hence in the formula for calculating the statistics value symbol $F$ appears (we calculate the variance relation in an analogous way as the F-test, with only other values distributions being measured). The definition of distribution between the groups and within the groups also becomes obvious.

The test name also becomes obvious, as it refers to the variance at the very moment the arithmetic mean values are compared. Calculating the number of the degrees of freedom (once referring to the number of classes – to determine the differences between the groups, and in the second case, to the total number – diminished by the number of the classes), also becomes evident.

Another example of using the ANOVA test is the case of looking for the differences between the mean values of the urine pH in groups composed according to the stone localization. The final decision after the conducted test is: there is no reason for the $H_0$ rejection. It signifies that there are no localization preferences that could be predicted upon the pH values in urine.[30]

Are we fully satisfied after the completion of the ANOVA test?
We have learnt that the differences between the mean values are statistically significant. Our curiosity prompts us another question: Which groups differ from one another, and which do not? There are several of them, and it happens to be more than a dozen of them. It is important, then, if the differences appeared for each couple, or if they apply only to several selected groups among the compared ones. The statistical packets are equipped with the procedures that answer our questions upon the subject. In case of the discussed SAS programme, such a procedure is the one of **Bonferroni**. The test belongs to the group of the so-called *post factum* tests (*post hoc*). The name suggests that they are performed after the previous finding of the differences with the ANOVA test.[31]
According to the notation assumed in the SAS programme, the results that inform us of the group couples between which the differences were found are marked with the asterisks in the table of results, in the right column (see the exercise step).
We can learn from the table which components of the stone can be predicted from the urine pH values, and which are impossible to differentiate on the basis of the analysis.
With the known urine pH, it is impossible to differentiate the xanthine – phosphate, the cistine – oxalate, the oxalate – uric acid, and the cistine – uric acid stones. The remaining "couples", in the light of the calculations made upon our data, can be differentiated on the urine pH value basis.

---

[30] A remark concerning the ANOVA test.
The ANOVA test, from the mathematical point of view, needs meeting many assumptions (meeting the assumption of the normal status of the distribution of the analyzed feature in all the compared groups is evident). One of the assumptions is the equality of variance in all the compared samples. It does not happen frequently that the required assumptions are met in the clinical data examination. Hence the test is performed without a particular condition analyzing, one should only be aware that the results obtained from the conducted ANOVA analysis should be very precisely justified with the mechanistic approach, that checks the results obtained in the context of more extensive knowledge upon the subject, or confirm the obtained results by a very detailed mechanistic approach, checking the obtained results in the context of a broader knowledge upon the subject, or confirm the results obtained with other calculating techniques. The opinion was taken from: Biostatistics, Wayne W. Daniel. P297. John Wiley & Sons New York, Chichester, Weinheim, Brisbane, Singapore, Toronto Seventh Edition 1999, Klaus Hinkelmann and Oscar Kempthorne, Design and Analysis of Experiments, Revised Edition, Wiley, New York, 1994, Douglas C. Montgomery, Design and Analysis of Experiments. Fourth Edition, Wiley, New York 1997, Jerome L. Myers and Arnold D. Well. Research Design and Statistical Analysis, Earlbaum Associates, Hillsdale, NJ 1995.
[31] The ANOVA test is reduced exactly to the F-test comparing the variances. An additional provision concerns only the ways of calculating the variance.

Answering the question asked at this step of analysis one should state, that no differences of the patients' bodily temperature have been found in the groups that resulted from the stone localization. So then, nothing can be concluded from the body temperature level about the deposit localization. However, the stone composition can be predicted upon the urine pH value. It is substantially meaningful for the further therapy. Defining the chemical composition of the stone is quite expensive, while marking the urine pH does not cause a financial problem. Hence, optimizing costs and benefits, one can base upon the pH test, predicting the stone composition and in the same way suggesting the therapeutic procedure.

In the summary of this part of the course, a general schedule of proceeding in inferential statistics which takes into account the sequence of performing the appropriate operations can be attached.

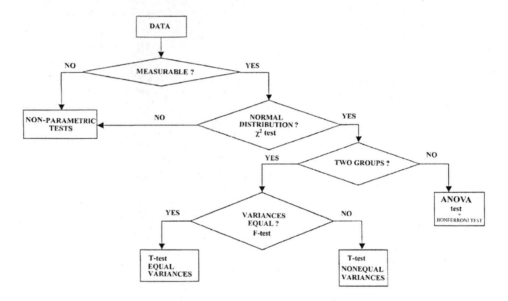

**Fig. 5.2.** An operation schedule in a complex statistical analysis depicting conditioning and relations among statistical tests

The schedule (Fig. 5.2.) depicts the sequence of the procedures performed depending on the fulfilment of conditions resulting primarily from the necessity of the distribution of normal character. As it can be seen in the schedule, using (applying) any of the **nonparametric tests (distribution free tests)** does not require any introductory conditions. The choice of the way compliant with the track called **parametric tests** is more favourable for the higher validity of those tests. In medical examination, the appearance of Gaussian distribution **(the parametric tests track)** is expected for the presence of the regulation systems, whose consequence is exactly a pretty frequent appearance of the normal distribution.

# Exercises

1. Conduct a comparative analysis of the impairment grade (expressed in %) in relation to the character in which the traffic accident casualty appeared (a cyclist, a pedestrian, etc.).
2. Ask a question of your own concerning the traffic accidents casualties' analysis, not forgetting either, that if any of the groups has a very low size (e.g. below 5 people) you should eliminate it from the analysis and explain if omitting the group can have a substantial impact on the analysis conducted.

# STEP 5 – exercise

# ANOVA test

---

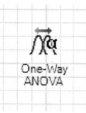

One-Way
ANOVA

A question is whether the pH of urine differs in groups with varying composition of urinary stones. In other words, do pH values predict which mineral crystallizes in the urinary tracts?

As usual we choose features to analyze; in this case it is the pH of urine and the main compound identified in the deposit. The pH is a measurable variable, whereas stone components are classical qualitative features (note the symbols next to the feature's names).

| ⊙ | pH | ♣ COMPOUND |
|---|---|---|
| | 7.3 | PHOSPHATE |
| | 5.2 | PHOSPHATE |
| | 6.9 | OXALATE |
| | 6.5 | PHOSPHATE |
| | 6.7 | OXALATE |
| | 5.6 | PHOSPHATE |
| | 6.1 | OXALATE |
| | 6.5 | OXALATE |
| | 6.4 | URICACID |
| | 5.7 | OXALATE |
| | 7.6 | OXALATE |
| | 5.7 | OXALATE |
| | 5.1 | PHOSPHATE |
| | 6.5 | OXALATE |
| | 6 | OXALATE |
| | 6.1 | OXALATE |

**Fig. 5.1.** Data fragment required for analysis. Patients will be divided according to stone composition, and the pH of urine will be analyzed

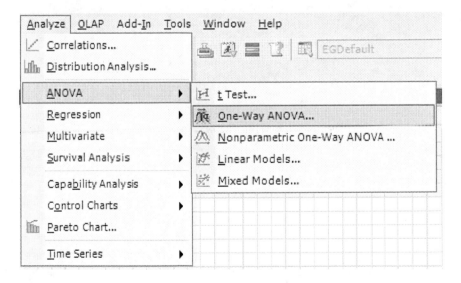

**Fig. 5.2.** Dialog box to select one-way ANOVA

ANOVA is selected as shown above. As in the example on t-test we define the role of each feature. The pH of urine is a measurable variable, whereas stone components are classical qualitative features. Urine pH values are grouped according to the main constituent of stones.

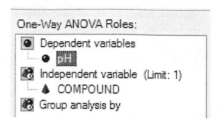

**Fig. 5.3.** Roles ascribed to variables (dependent variable – pH, independent variable – division into groups – compound)

As you know SAS is a professional and very complete package. Do not be surprised if you have to answer a number of questions when choosing the program version. In the next dialog box we choose a test (for instance Welch's variance-weighted ANOVA) and Levene's test (homogeneity of variances).

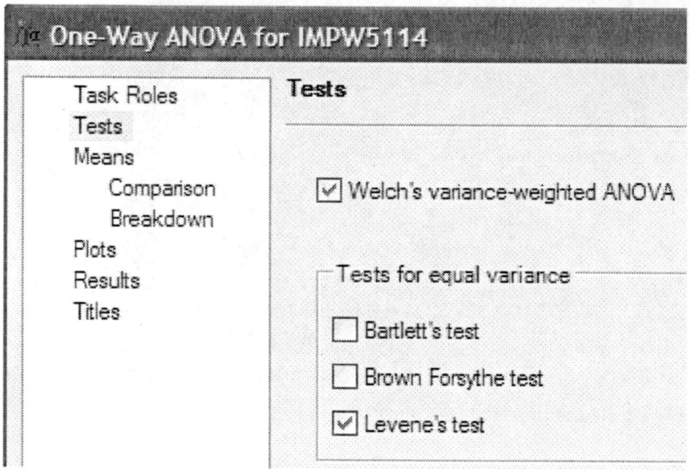

**Fig. 5.4.** You select the version of ANOVA and a test for equal variance. ANOVA should be used only for comparison of groups with equal variances (Levene's test)

We said before that it is not enough to know that pH values differ in groups (stone composition). There are several groups and it is interesting to find out which pair of groups differs or not. Bonferroni test is used to carry out pairwise comparisons. You select the test (in a long list of tests) and define the confidence level in the next dialog box (Fig. 5.5.).

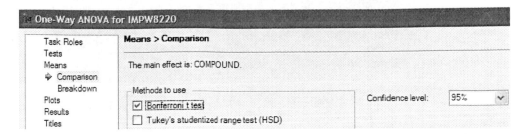

**Fig. 5.5.** Select post hoc Bonferroni test option to carry out pair-wise comparisons of the group mean

In the dialog box below tick the statistics for quantitative variables, taking into account division into groups.

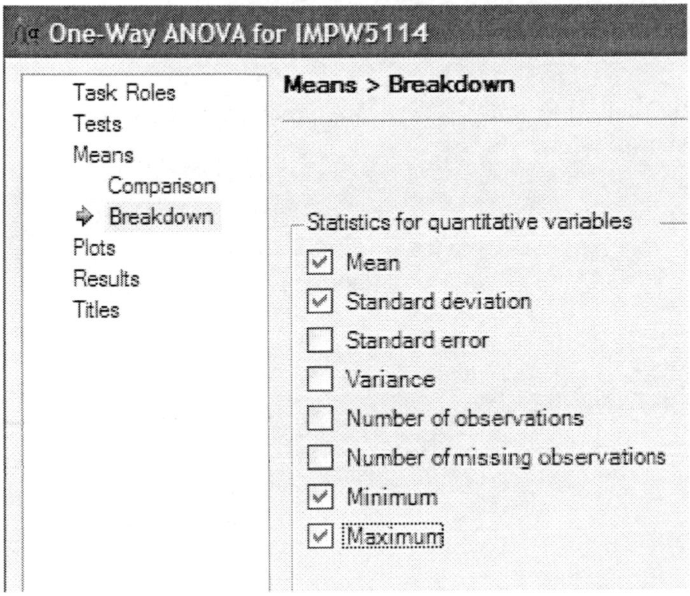

**Fig. 5.6.** Parameters that describe the groups

The familiar dialog box to specify graphic options to display the results is available also in ANOVA procedure.

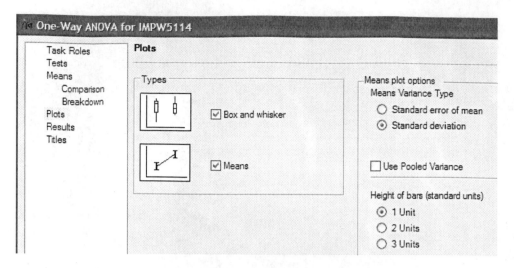

**Fig. 5.7.** Selection of graphic options to display the results

Click the "Run" button to start the ANOVA procedure. Results of one-way analysis of variance are shown below.

### One-Way Analysis of Variance
### Results

### *The ANOVA Procedure*

| Class Level Information | | |
|---|---|---|
| **Class** | **Levels** | **Values** |
| COMPOUND | 5 | CYS XANT OXALATE PHOSPHATE URICACID |

**Fig. 5.8.** Table provides the number and names of groups (divided by qualitative features – stone composition)

Remember (see the questionnaire) that analysis of stone composition revealed the presence of five main constituents. The number of identified classes reminds us of this fact (the program found five different terms in column "COMPOUND"). It is important to be cautious and precise when coding or entering the names of qualitative variables. If you make a mistake and write "URIACID" instead of "URICACID" the system identifies a new group and patients would be divided in the wrong way.

| Number of Observations Read | 269 |
|---|---|
| Number of Observations Used | 256 |

**Fig. 5.9.** Table provides sample size (those who have only one of two features are excluded from analysis)

The table above informs us that the program found 256 records with two results (pH of urine and the main constituent of crystalline deposit).

One-Way Analysis of Variance
Results

The ANOVA Procedure

Dependent Variable: pH

| Source | DF | Sum of Squares | Mean Square | F Value | Pr > F |
|---|---|---|---|---|---|
| Model | 4 | 156.6956122 | 39.1739031 | 462.89 | <.0001 |
| Error | 251 | 21.2418878 | 0.0846290 | | |
| Corrected Total | 255 | 177.9375000 | | | |

| R-Square | Coeff Var | Root MSE | pH Mean |
|---|---|---|---|
| 0.880622 | 4.675611 | 0.290911 | 6.221875 |

**Fig. 5.10.** Table providing the degrees of freedom, sums of squares, F values and p value which is very low, meaning that inter-group differences are significant

The table above resembles the table inserted in the theoretical part of the book, only the terms used may be slightly different ("Model" – instead of "inter-group relations" and "Error" – instead of "intra-group relations"). Degrees of freedom, sums of squares and mean squares are the same as in the theoretical part of the book. F values and p values are provided in the last two columns. The very low p value indicates that $H_0$ should be rejected, which means that the difference in mean pH between groups identified by the main stone constituent is significant.

# One-Way Analysis of Variance
## Results

*The ANOVA Procedure*

| Levene's Test for Homogeneity of pH Variance ANOVA of Squared Deviations from Group Means | | | | | |
|---|---|---|---|---|---|
| Source | DF | Sum of Squares | Mean Square | F Value | Pr > F |
| COMP# | 3 | 1.0452 | 0.3484 | 17.39 | <.0001 |
| Error | 250 | 5.0098 | 0.0200 | | |

| Welch's ANOVA for pH | | | |
|---|---|---|---|
| Source | DF | F Value | Pr > F |
| COMP# | 4.0000 | 589.02 | <.0001 |
| Error | 6.1207 | | |

**Fig. 5.11.** Tables with results

Results obtained by use of Levene's test and Welch's test confirm the concordance between the results of the three tests (low p values, which in statistics always mean that $H_0$ should be rejected).

| Level of COMP# | N | pH | |
|---|---|---|---|
| | | Mean | Std Dev |
| CYS | 4 | 5.72500000 | 0.86168440 |
| XANT | 2 | 7.20000000 | 0.14142136 |
| OXALATE | 147 | 5.80680272 | 0.30580231 |
| PHOSPHATE | 61 | 7.60000000 | 0.19407902 |
| URICACID | 42 | 5.67380952 | 0.27413680 |

**Fig. 5.12.** Table with parameters of each stone constituent

A measures of location (arithmetic mean) and dispersion (standard deviation) for pH value in each group separately are obtained separately.

| Comparisons significant at the 0.05 level are indicated by ***. | | | | |
|---|---|---|---|---|
| COMP# Comparison | Difference Between Means | Simultaneous 95% Confidence Limits | | |
| PHOSPHATE - XANT | 0.40000 | -0.19204 | 0.99204 | |
| PHOSPHATE - OXALATE | 1.79320 | 1.66772 | 1.91868 | *** |
| PHOSPHATE - CYS | 1.87500 | 1.44977 | 2.30023 | *** |
| PHOSPHATE - URICACID | 1.92619 | 1.76100 | 2.09138 | *** |
| XANT - PHOSPHATE | -0.40000 | -0.99204 | 0.19204 | |
| XANT - OXALATE | 1.39320 | 0.80668 | 1.97972 | *** |
| XANT - CYS | 1.47500 | 0.76150 | 2.18850 | *** |
| XANT - URICACID | 1.52619 | 0.92991 | 2.12247 | *** |
| OXALATE - PHOSPHATE | -1.79320 | -1.91868 | -1.66772 | *** |
| OXALATE - XANT | -1.39320 | -1.97972 | -0.80668 | *** |
| OXALATE - CYS | 0.08180 | -0.33570 | 0.49931 | |
| OXALATE - URICACID | 0.13299 | -0.01116 | 0.27714 | |
| CYS - PHOSPHATE | -1.87500 | -2.30023 | -1.44977 | *** |

**Fig. 5.13.a.** Pair-wise differences between means. Three asterisks in the right column denote a statistically significant difference

| | | | |
|---|---|---|---|
| OXALATE - PHOSPHATE | -1.79320 | -1.91868 | -1.66772 | *** |
| OXALATE - XANT | -1.39320 | -1.97972 | -0.80668 | *** |
| OXALATE - CYS | 0.08180 | -0.33570 | 0.49931 | |
| OXALATE - URICACID | 0.13299 | -0.01116 | 0.27714 | |
| CYS - PHOSPHATE | -1.87500 | -2.30023 | -1.44977 | *** |
| CYS - XANT | -1.47500 | -2.18850 | -0.76150 | *** |
| CYS - OXALATE | -0.08180 | -0.49931 | 0.33570 | |
| CYS - URICACID | 0.05119 | -0.37992 | 0.48230 | |
| URICACID - PHOSPHATE | -1.92619 | -2.09138 | -1.76100 | *** |
| URICACID - XANT | -1.52619 | -2.12247 | -0.92991 | *** |
| URICACID - OXALATE | -0.13299 | -0.27714 | 0.01116 | |
| URICACID - CYS | -0.05119 | -0.48230 | 0.37992 | |

**Fig. 5.13.b.** Continuation – Pair-wise differences between means. Three asterisks in the right column denote a statistically significant difference

The table shows all pair-wise comparisons among arithmetic means and identifies pairs of means which differ significantly (three asterisks in the right column), and simultaneously provides the results of Bonferroni procedure. The first column lists the differences between means whereas the second and third columns list the lower and upper 95% confidence limits, meaning that there is a 95% probability that a similar result would occur in our database if the study was repeated in another population.

| COMP# | Mean of pH | Std. Dev. of pH | Variance of pH | Minimum of pH | Maximum of pH |
|---|---|---|---|---|---|
| | 6.22188 | 0.83534 | 0.69779 | 5.0 | 7.9 |
| CYS | 5.72500 | 0.86168 | 0.74250 | 5.2 | 7.0 |
| XANT | 7.20000 | 0.14142 | 0.02000 | 7.1 | 7.3 |
| OXALATE | 5.80680 | 0.30580 | 0.09352 | 5.1 | 6.8 |
| PHOSPHATE | 7.60000 | 0.19408 | 0.03767 | 7.1 | 7.9 |
| URICACID | 5.67381 | 0.27414 | 0.07515 | 5.0 | 6.1 |

**Fig. 5.14.** Parameters that describe pH in various groups

Note that CYS and XANT groups are small (see table above). Statistics – a part of mathematics developing tools for analysis of large datasets, does not like small sample sizes. In order to make more accurate generalizations, it is advisable to exclude patients with very rare observations.

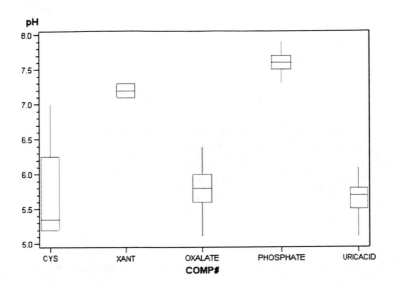

**Fig. 5.15.** Graphic display of the results. Box and whisker plots

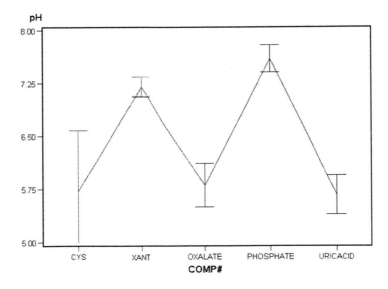

**Fig. 5.16.** Another type of graphic display of the results

138

These two plots are self-explanatory and no comment or interpretation is required. The relation between groups is clearly visible.

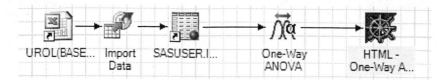

UROL(BASE...   Import   SASUSER.I...        One-Way        HTML -
              Data                      ANOVA     One-Way A...

**Fig. 5.17.** Representation of the process in ANOVA calculation

Analysis carried out in the calculation process assumes the form as shown above (Fig. 5.17.).

As already mentioned it is purposeful to eliminate small samples. Individual records can be excluded from reporting using "Filter Data" option on the dropdown Data menu.

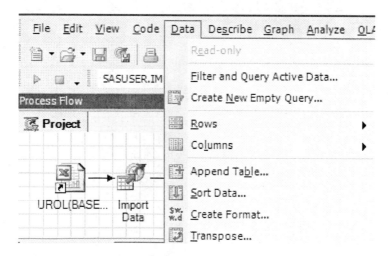

**Fig. 5.18.** Data filtering to exclude subjects with CYS and XANT stone components (too small samples)

After choosing Filter Data you define the conditions of record exclusion in a new dialog box. In this example you eliminate records which contain CYS and XANT in the column Compound. The exclusion of records containing CYS is illustrated below. We should comment briefly on the Operator box. It provides a scrolldown menu containing a long list of options. If you eliminate records according to numerical criteria, the operator will assume the form of mathematical expression. In this example you exclude records according to text criteria and therefore you use the "equals" option and write CYS in parentheses to denote it is a text symbol.

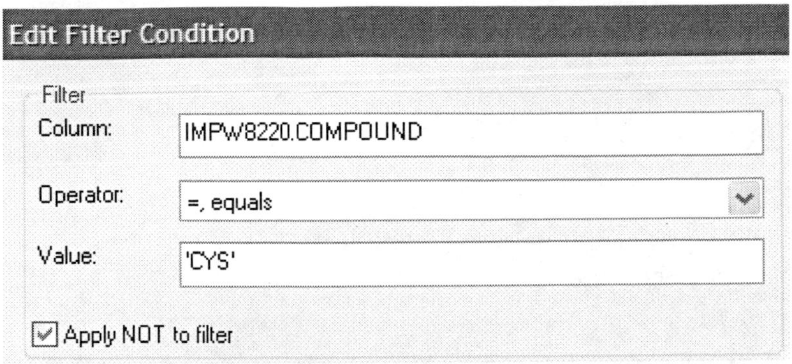

**Edit Filter Condition**

Filter
Column: IMPW8220.COMPOUND

Operator: =, equals

Value: 'CYS'

☑ Apply NOT to filter

**Fig. 5.19.** Defining the conditions of record elimination (CYS and XANT are text symbols and we use the „equals" option)

As you see, there is a tick next to "Apply NOT to filer". It means that records do NOT having "CYS" will remain in the set. If you forget to tick this option, your database will contain the records with "CYS". The details of filtering procedure were shown in STEP 3.

An identical filtering procedure referring to records containing "XANT" is applied to eliminate subjects with xanthine as the main stone component. As expected, we obtain the final table with only three groups identified by the program.

**One-Way Analysis of Variance**
**Results**

*The ANOVA Procedure*

| Class Level Information | | |
|---|---|---|
| Class | Levels | Values |
| COMP# | 3 | OXALATE PHOSPHATE URICACID |

| Number of Observations Read | 250 |
|---|---|
| Number of Observations Used | 250 |

**Fig. 5.20.** Tables with the identified groups without CYS and XANT groups

As you may see, the number of observations is also reduced.

*Dependent Variable: pH*

| Source | DF | Sum of Squares | Mean Square | F Value | Pr > F |
|---|---|---|---|---|---|
| Model | 2 | 153.7946122 | 76.8973061 | 999.96 | <.0001 |
| Error | 247 | 18.9943878 | 0.0769004 | | |
| Corrected Total | 249 | 172.7890000 | | | |

**Fig. 5.21.** Tables containing the results of calculations. The value of statistics F and *"p"* value suggests rejection of $H_0$

The results summarized in the table remain unchanged. The final result, suggesting us to reject $H_0$, remains unchanged because of the very low p value. There are some differences when it comes to the details after exclusion of some records, but it does not affect the final result.

| Levene's Test for Homogeneity of pH Variance ANOVA of Squared Deviations from Group Means | | | | | |
|---|---|---|---|---|---|
| Source | DF | Sum of Squares | Mean Square | F Value | Pr > F |
| COMP# | 2 | 0.1347 | 0.0674 | 4.82 | 0.0089 |
| Error | 247 | 3.4531 | 0.0140 | | |

| Welch's ANOVA for pH | | | |
|---|---|---|---|
| Source | DF | F Value | Pr > F |
| COMP# | 2.0000 | 1531.44 | <.0001 |
| Error | 105.2 | | |

**Fig. 5.22.** Results of the tests

The results obtained from the Welch's and Levene's tests imply that $H_0$ should be rejected.

| Level of COMP# | N | pH | |
| | | Mean | Std Dev |
|---|---|---|---|
| OXALATE | 147 | 5.80680272 | 0.30580231 |
| PHOSPHATE | 61 | 7.60000000 | 0.19407902 |
| URICACID | 42 | 5.67380952 | 0.27413680 |

**Fig. 5.23.** Descriptive statistics for the three groups

Descriptive statistics for the remaining groups remains unchanged.

## One-Way Analysis of Variance Results

### The ANOVA Procedure

### Bonferroni (Dunn) t Tests for pH

**Fig. 5.24.** Caption of the Bonferroni procedure

| Comparisons significant at the 0.05 level are indicated by ***. | | | | |
|---|---|---|---|---|
| COMP# Comparison | Difference Between Means | Simultaneous 95% Confidence Limits | | |
| PHOSPHATE - OXALATE | 1.79320 | 1.69139 | 1.89500 | *** |
| PHOSPHATE - URICACID | 1.92619 | 1.79217 | 2.06021 | *** |
| OXALATE - PHOSPHATE | -1.79320 | -1.89500 | -1.69139 | *** |
| OXALATE - URICACID | 0.13299 | 0.01604 | 0.24994 | *** |
| URICACID - PHOSPHATE | -1.92619 | -2.06021 | -1.79217 | *** |
| URICACID - OXALATE | -0.13299 | -0.24994 | -0.01604 | *** |

**Fig. 5.25.** Results of Bonferroni post hoc pair-wise comparison test show significant differences in the mean pH of urine between groups identified according to stone composition

The table summarizing the results of the Bonferroni procedure remains unchanged except number of rows.

| COMP# | Mean of pH | Std. Dev. of pH | Variance of pH | Minimum of pH | Maximum of pH |
|-------|-----------|-----------------|----------------|---------------|---------------|
|  | 6.22200 | 0.83303 | 0.69393 | 5.0 | 7.9 |
| OXALATE | 5.80680 | 0.30580 | 0.09352 | 5.1 | 6.8 |
| PHOSPHATE | 7.60000 | 0.19408 | 0.03767 | 7.1 | 7.9 |
| URICACID | 5.67381 | 0.27414 | 0.07515 | 5.0 | 6.1 |

**Fig. 5.26.** Descriptive statistics of the groups included in analysis

Description of other groups included in analysis remains unchanged.

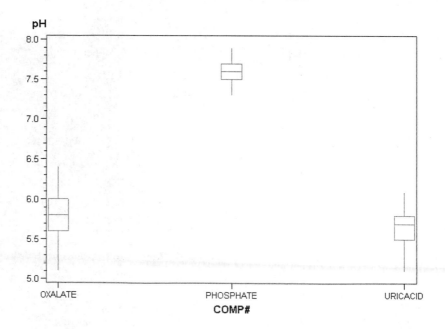

**Fig. 5.27.** Graphic display of the results

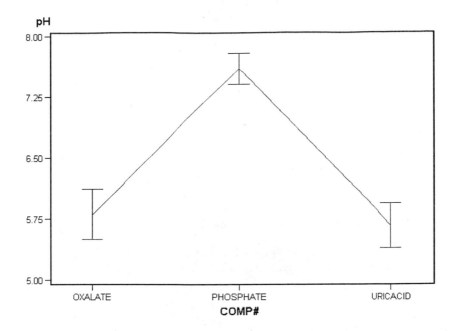

**Fig. 5.28.** Another type of graphic display of the results

The only difference between the plots is the number of groups for comparison.

Two more steps have been added to the list of procedures. The process of filtering is denoted by an icon „Query". Each time you modify your database (in this example – filtering) a new version of the data is obtained (SASUSER). The ANOVA procedure was applied only when filtering had been performed twice.

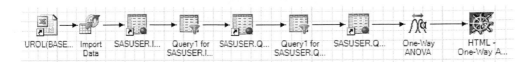

**Fig. 5.29.** Representation of the process in ANOVA calculation with double data filtering (exclusion of records coded as CYS and XANT)

A symbol of the result set appears at the end.

If you want to continue analysis using the complete database, click on the icon "UROL(BASE...". If you activate the first icon "SASUSER.Q...", calculations are done using the modified database without records coded as "CYS" in the column "COMPOUND".

# STEP 6

## Correlation and regression
## Are any variables mutually dependent?

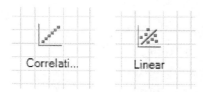

Correlati...    Linear

> **Is there any relationship between the urine pH and the urine density?**
> **Can we predict the probable stone composition on the basis of the known value of urine pH and its unit weight?**

Search for the correlation (interrelation between the measurable features) may be expressed by two characteristics: correlation coefficient value, which measures the strength of the association between two variables and the regression analysis that characterises the type of the relation (the linear, hyperbolic, parabolic or, perhaps another one type of dependency).[32] A very simple urine analysis may be performed by measuring its pH and its density. These are inexpensive tests and for that reason commonly performed. Can we obtain information about the illness background from the mutual relation between those two features in a nephrolithiasis case?

It should be pointed out that both features are measurable the analysis of which is usually started with presenting the results, in the form of so called scatter plot to display these values put into the Cartesian coordinates system. Each point has the value of one variable determining its position on the horizontal axis (X-axis) and the value of the

---

[32] The scope of this book encompasses only the linear relation. The other ones have been enumerated only for the sake of awareness of a great possible relation types variety between the features.

second feature on the vertical axis (*Y*-axis). The distribution of the points representing the results in our sample where e.g. the *X*-axis represents the urine density, while the *Y*-axis the urine pH values is shown in Fig. 6.1.[33]

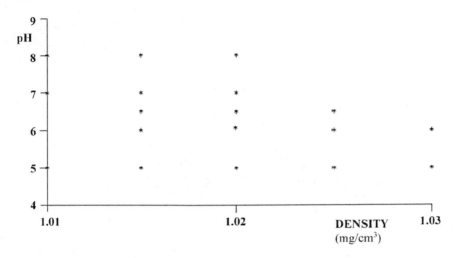

**Fig. 6.1.** Urine pH as dependent on the urine density (unit weight)

A visual interpretation of the illustration obtained can tell us a lot about the relation between the two measurable features – in our case between the pH values and the values expressing urine specific gravity.

First of all, one should realize exactly that each point represents two values (in our example, pH and the specific gravity) describing the same person. It is very important that these two values represent the analysis results of the same urine sample.[34] The scatter plot as we expect can be very varied. The points can be arranged along one straight line (a very strong dependence) or around an another curve (in mathematics line is also a curve), but they can also be spread all over the area between the *X*-and *Y*-axes of the coordinate system (no relation). In our example, the distribution is pretty large. If someone judged by the surface of the area taken by the points one could think that there is no relation (no correlation) between the analysed features.

It is only our subjective estimate, though. The objective decision can be taken applying particular tests to validate the significance of two kinds of the relation characteristics:

---

[33] Very frequently, analyzing an unfamiliar problem, we cannot specify the given feature status as an independent or dependent. All the same we could assume that the *X*-axis represents the urine pH, and the *Y*-axis its specific density. Only on the basis of analyzing the supposed mechanism responsible for the system observed is it possible to ascribe a role in the mutual arrangement of both analyzed features.

[34] If only one of the two markings was done with a given person, the result is excluded from the dependence analysis. Program automatically eliminates incomplete results.

Two methods are available:

1. Calculating the correlation coefficient – "$r$";
2. Setting the regression function (here we are going to discuss only the linear regression) $y = ax + b$ [35].

The correlation coefficient expresses the strength of the two features mutual dependence.

The correlation coefficient $r$ value is contained in the range from –1 to 1. [36]

The correlation coefficient for the linear dependence is expressed with the following formula:

$$r = \frac{n\sum x_i y_i - \left(\sum x_i\right)\left(\sum y_i\right)}{\sqrt{n\sum x_i^2 - \left(\sum x_i\right)^2}\sqrt{n\sum y_i^2 - \left(\sum y_i\right)^2}}$$  (eq. 6.1.)

In our example this value equals –0.33.

The value of correlation coefficient, as it has been told above, is contained in the range from –1 to +1. The closer to zero is its value, the weaker the dependence is. If it equals zero it signifies that we do not state any dependence. The closer to +1 or –1 its value is, the stronger dependence we state between the analysed features. What makes the value positive or negative? If along with the increase of one feature's value, the other one grows, too, it signifies that the features are directly proportional to each other and the value $r$ of the correlation coefficient is positive. The increase of one feature's value accompanied by the decreases of the second variable signifies that the features are inversely proportional. The correlation coefficient assumes negative values then. Thus we know, that in our case the inverse proportion relation appears. Interpreting the correlation coefficient absolute value one could think that the relation is not statistically significant. It is only our subjective estimate, though. We shall obtain an objective evaluation if we perform an appropriate statistical test that will determine the correlation coefficient significance.

Another type of dependence analysis is looking for the so-called regression function. If our collection of points observed in an empirical way can be presented as a certain precisely defined line and that line can be recorded as an appropriate mathematical function, then this function will be specified as the function of regression (examples of other, nonlinear regression functions will be presented in the further part of this hand-

---

[35] Exactly the regression model takes the element of randomisation into account. This is why the precise function takes the form: $y = ax + b + \varepsilon$ where $\varepsilon$ represents the effects of the influence on any additional random parameters. To make this manual easy for non-professionalists, this aspect will not be discusses in this manual.

[36] The frame of this course encompasses only the linear relation, hence only this case will be discussed thoroughly. The examples of nonlinear dependence will be discussed only qualitatively.

book). There are special procedures[37] that enable making the right choice of function and calculate all the parameters of a given function.
The linear function notation:

$$\hat{y} = ax + b,$$ (eq. 6.2.)

where $x$ signifies the value that is assumed by the feature recognized as the independent variable (urine density), $a$ and $b$ are the linear function parameters (their values are appointed for each set of points), while $y$ – the dependent variable (the circumflex over the symbol $y$ signifies the value defined according to the equation) expresses the pH of urine.

The specific linear function will be found if we learn the values of $a$ and $b$ parameters. The method of least squares mentioned in the footnote[38] provides the formulae for calculating both parameters.

$$a = \frac{\sum_{i=1}^{n}(x_i - \overline{x})(y_i - \overline{y})}{\sum_{i=1}^{n}(x_i - \overline{x})^2} = \frac{\sum_{i=1}^{n}x_i y_i - n\overline{x}\,\overline{y}}{\sum_{i=1}^{n}x_i^2 - n\overline{x}^2}, \qquad b = \overline{y} - a\overline{x},$$ (eq. 6.3.)

where the symbols with circumflex signify the appropriate values of arithmetic mean values.

The linear function of regression found by us assumes the graphically presented form as in Fig. 6.2.

---

[37] The most popular is the method called "least squares method" which takes the sum of shortest distances (in squares) versus the observed point and the expected point calculated according to the regression function form. There are two unknown values (parameters: "a" and "b"). The set of two equations makes possible calculating the values of these two parameters.
[38] The least squares method is of general character and may be applied to any kind of function not limited to linear function exclusively.

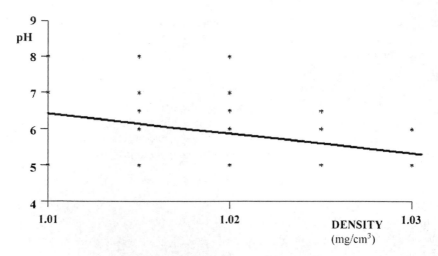

**Fig. 6.2.** The dependence of urine specific gravity on the pH of urine, along with the appointed function of linear regression

The regression function notation for our example assumes the following form:

$$pH(ourY) = -452.49D(ourX) + 467.87 \qquad \text{(eq. 6.4.)}$$

where D signifies the urine density.

As it can be seen, the slope coefficient calculated for our example has a negative value. It signifies that the function is the decreasing one. The higher the urine specific gravity the lower is its pH value. The minus symbol of the slope coefficient $a$ remains in a strict connection with the correlation coefficient value $r$, that is also negative.

The dispersion of points needs several more comments:
1. Two features persuaded visualize the issues discussed in the first chapter. Both the specific gravity and the pH value are continuous and measurable features. The discrete character of values is clearly visible in the illustration, and it results exactly from the measuring instruments precision.
2. The next remark is a direct consequence of the first one. It should not be forgotten that there are over 150 people in our group (the aforesaid markings were not made with each and every patient). The number of points in the illustration is much lower than the patients' number, which results from the fact that both measurements were made for the smaller number of people (missing data). It results also from the doubling of several points, and the number of people represented by the given point is unknown.
   If each point represented only one person, the regression function would assume (and perhaps it would have assumed) a different shape.

We have calculated the value of correlation coefficient and the shape of the linear regression function. A question still remains, whether these values are significant, as we do not know which value of the correlation coefficient should be neglected and which should be treated as significant.

For that purpose, we apply two tests:

1. Correlation coefficient significance test;
2. Regression coefficient significance test.

Testing procedures are compatible with already assumed schedule.

1. $H_0$ – correlation coefficient $r = 0$ there is no dependence between the analysed features.
   $H_1$ – correlation coefficient $r <> 0$ there is dependence between the analysed features.

2. Degrees of freedom number

$$df = n - 2. \qquad \text{(eq. 6.5.)}$$

   The significance level (assumed) $\alpha$

3. The statistics value:

$$t = r\sqrt{\frac{n-2}{1-r^2}} \qquad \text{(eq. 6.6.)}$$

   where: $n$ – number of cases, $r$ – correlation coefficient.

4. The "p" – value appropriate for $t$ value

5. The final decision: "p" $< \alpha$ – $H_0$ is rejected;

   "p" $> \alpha$ – there are no grounds to reject $H_0$.

6. Interpretation.

In our case (detailed calculations were presented in the workbook part) we state that the correlation coefficient is statistically significant, which we would not probably find out upon the sole visual estimation.

The procedure of testing the significance of the slope coefficient ($a$) of the linear function is the following:

1. $H_0$ – the directional coefficient is not significant.
   The directional coefficient is equal zero[33].

   $H_1$ – there is a dependence between the analysed features.

2. The degrees of freedom number.

   $df = n - 2$

   The significance level (assumed) $\alpha$

3. The statistics value:

$$t = \frac{a - \alpha_0}{s_r} \sqrt{\sum_{i=1}^{n} (x_i - \bar{x})^2} \; , \qquad \text{(eq. 6.7.)}$$

where: $\quad s_r = \sqrt{\dfrac{\sum_{i=1}^{n} (y_i - \hat{y}_i)^2}{n - 2}} \; ;$

$\hat{y}_i$ – theoretical value for the given $x_i$,
$a$ – the directional coefficient value,
$\alpha_0$ – the directional coefficient value (especially 0), in relation to which we differences.

4. The read value "p".

5. The final decision: "p" $< \alpha$ – $H_0$ is rejected:

   "p" $> \alpha$ – there are no grounds for the rejection of $H_0$.

6. Interpretation.

### Interpretation

In our example we have found both the significance of the correlation coefficient (despite its relatively low absolute value), and the significance of the directional coefficient of the linear function. We can state, then, that the specific gravity remains in the statistically significant relation inversely proportional to the urine pH value.

> **NOTA BENE**
> Neither the correlation coefficient significance nor the significance of the regression function depend on the variable character: dependent and independent. For the reverse arrangement (the substantial gravity as dependent on pH) the statistics values would be different, but the final decision appears be the same (also significant).

The very statement that there is a significant dependence between the features does not indicate the mechanism that would explain the appointed relation. So the further question concerns the mechanism that leads to such a significant dependence.

Another question also appears, if it has anything in common with the urine composition, as we would like to make use of those simple markings in order to foresee what kind of stone we are dealing with in a given case.

We shall find the answer to this question when we have performed another analysis, that applies to studying the certain processes' mechanism and is not directly connected with our questionnaire and the data collected from the patients.

In order to find the answer to our question, if the urine density can result from different solubility of particular salts, we shall test the salts' solubility depending on the urine pH value. If such a dependence explained the above obtained result of the significant dependence between the urine pH value and its density it would signify, that we can foresee excessive concentrations of the relevant salts, and in the next stage a possible deposit composition.

The results of the laboratory tests aimed at the specification of the maximum concentrations of the given salt in the solution of the specific pH value are shown in Fig. 6.3.

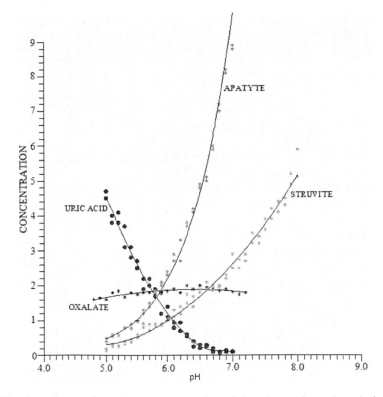

**Fig. 6.3.** The dependence of maximum concentration of the given salt on the solution pH value (struvite and apatite are phosphate salts)

The regression functions[39] have been calculated for those experimental points (the measurements are multiple and the results can differ from one another). This time, as it can be seen, in no case is it a straight line (the linear regression function). Below, the forms of functions that represent the given points for each compound have been introduced (applying also the least-square method):

**URIC ACID – the 6-th degree polynominal**

$$Y = -0.9288 * x^6 + 33.35 * x^5 - 497.58 * x^4 + 3947.7 * x^3 - 17566.2 * x^2 + 41560.2 * x - 40830.6 \qquad \text{(eq. 6.8.)}$$

**OXALATE – the 2-nd degree polynominal**

$$Y = -0.1126 * x^2 + 1.44 * x - 2.715 \qquad \text{(eq. 6.9.)}$$

**APATITE – the exponential function**

$$Y = 0.000272728 * \exp(1.499 * x) \qquad \text{(eq. 6.10.)}$$

**STRUVITE the 2-nd degree polynominal**

$$Y = 0.4635 * x^2 - 4.41 * x + 10.78, \qquad \text{(eq. 6.11.)}$$

where $Y$ signifies the suitable salt concentration (mmol/l), while $x$ signifies the solution pH value.

As it can be seen in this example, the form of regression (approximation) function can sometimes be very complicated. It is important that this function's form adequately represents the points distribution.

There are many methods to transform the non-linear regression function into the linear form (for example introducing the logarithmic scale for some variables) to apply the complete analysis of mutual relation between particular variables (calculation and estimation of correlation coefficient as well as linear function parameters and their significance).

Apatite and struvite are phosphate salts and they were both treated jointly in our questionnaire.

In order to explain all the conditioning, one should know the molecular mass of the analysed salts (they are given in the following table).

---

[39] The regression functions in this specific case are also called approximation functions, which is more a mathematical than a statistical term.

| MOLECULAR MASS (g) | CHEMICAL COMPOUND |
|---|---|
| 128 | OXYLATES |
| 137 | PHOSPHATE – STRUVITE |
| 165 | URINE ACID |
| 295 | PHOSPHATE – APATITE |

**Tab. 6.1.** Molecular masses of the discussed salts

Did the conducted analysis help us foresee the kind of salt upon the knowledge of urine pH and specific gravity values?

If the high solubility of the salts like apatite or struvite (and their high content in urine), which grows with the urine alkalinity, was responsible for the increase of the urine gravity, we should have observed a reverse situation in our previous analysis, which is to say the directly proportional dependence of the urine specific gravity of its pH value. This is not the case, though.

Our answer to the question if we can conclude anything about the urine composition upon the measurement of its gravity and pH (obviously, from the aspect of salts that are interesting to us for their crystallization) is NO. The compound that shows a similar dependence is uric acid. If this compound was exclusively responsible for the urine specific gravity, we could conclude the presence of this solution in urine. It should be pointed out that this salt has the lowest specific gravity out of all the salts considered. That way it cannot compete with the salts, whose solubility grows with the urine pH value. Moreover, these salts have a very high specific gravity (compared to uric acid). (Tab. 6.1.). Other components that influence urine specific gravity along with the urine pH increase (alkalization) are visible. Perhaps high specific gravity results from the presence of compounds that are metabolism products. Confirming that supposition would require a further study, but in our example we discuss only the pH relation to the salts that are present in urine.

Stating the presence and defining the dependence form (the regression function form) and the correlation coefficient does not exhaust the subject. As a rule, it is only the first step in the dependence analysis among the features studied.

We have found that the dependence between the specific gravity and the urine pH is statistically significant. In spite of performing additional tests, we did not manage to find the mechanism of this phenomenon. Perhaps we would find the justification for this observation following the further analyses.

Looking for the mechanisms responsible for the observed dependencies, one should consider the following models:

$$X \Rightarrow Y,$$

where $Y$ value is a direct result of a given value of $X$ feature:

$$X_1 \Rightarrow X_2 \Rightarrow X_3 \Rightarrow \ldots \ldots \Rightarrow X_i \Rightarrow \ldots \ldots \Rightarrow Y,$$

where *Y* value is the final result of the sequence of many transformations and intermediate stages,

$$X \searrow \quad \nearrow Y$$
$$Z$$

where the values *X* and *Y* are not mutually related, but constitute the joint effect of the
presence of an unknown feature *Z*, that manages (influences) both the *X* and *Y* features.
Finding the intermediate stages or the common factor presence can be specified as
recognizing the mechanism responsible for the dependence observed.
The most frequently discovered mechanism represents an arrangement composed of all
the enumerated dependence forms.

One more remark concerning the regression function analysis results which are presented in the SAS programme result window.

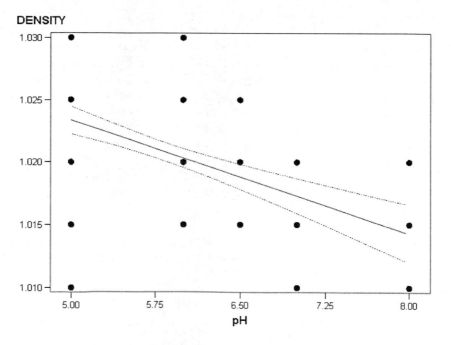

**Fig. 6.4.** The result of the regression function calculations made in SAS packet (with the marked
confidence range option is presented in detail in the workbook part)

As it can be seen in Fig. 6.4. apart from the linear regression function, two other
(dashed) curves were shown at its both sides. It is a good moment to return to the already learnt before notion of confidence interval. The regression function form depends largely on the experimental points distributions. The appointed linear function of

regression certainly is not the line for the population, but for the sample. It is obvious that if the set of conditions was changed, automatically the regression function would change its position in the coordinate system. In statistics, we must be constantly aware of this fact. The appointed area, specified as the confidence interval (or prediction interval) for the regression function is to meet this uncertainty (see the workbook). The area appointed by two dashed lines specifies the range in which fall the predicted values of a dependent variable with a 95% probability. The shape of the lines that define the confidence interval results also from the multiplicity of particular points (which is not visible in the illustration, although taken into account in calculations).

### The outliers (outstanding points)

The problem of outliers has already been discussed before, in the context of the measured variable distribution. This time we shall discuss the problem of outliers in the regression analysis. Fig. 6.5. shows dependence between the hemoglobin concentration (production) in the patient's blood and the erythrocyte number in the microscope picture of blood. The regression function for the whole set was drawn as the red line. Removing the outliers (distinguished by the ellipses) causes the regression function assume the shape as shown with the blue line. As it has already been said, removing the set elements equals removing the patient from the analysed sample. This is not allowed. However, if there are measurements, that are evidently contrary to the general trend, they can be removed, provided the precise definition of membership criterion in the group excluded from the further analysis.

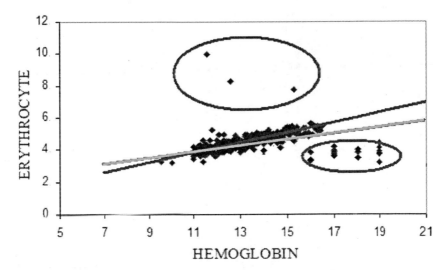

**Fig. 6.5.** The outliers in the regression analysis. It was shown that a few points that depart from the general trend may cause the different final results of the regression analysis. The examination of the distribution points in the coordinate arrangement is important for the analysis correctness

156

The function equation for all the observations:

$$Erythr. = 0.1187 * Hemogl + 2.79 \qquad \text{(eq. 6.12.)}$$

The regression equation for the sample after the exclusion

$$Erythr. = 0.2747 * Hemogl + 0.844 \qquad \text{(eq. 6.13.)}$$

Why could we temporarily remove the marked results from the analysis?
The top ellipse marks the people with anaemia caused by the iron deficiency. The bottom ellipse marks the people with high B12 avitaminosis. With the known criteria of eliminating people from the analysis we can state, that the relation between the haemoglobin concentration and the erythrocyte number is expressed by eq. 6.13., although the relation between those two features of the analysed sample is expressed with eq. 6.12.

More detailed information concerning the regression analysis is given in the footnote[40] for the Reader interested in mathematical aspects of this analysis.

---

[40] There are many assumptions which are expected to be satisfied by the distribution of the empirical points. The most important is the dependent variable to represent the normal distribution for each value of independent variable. It is visualized in Fig. 6F. The positions of mean values of dependent variable for each independent variable determine the position of regression function. The collection of data shall take into account this type of conditions to make the analysis reliable.

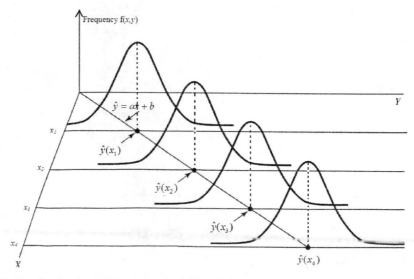

**Fig. 6.F.** The distribution of dependent variable ($Y$) for selected values of independent variable ($X$). The averaged values of $Y$ (maximum frequency) for particular $X$-value determines the position of theoretical linear regression function

# Exercises

1. Ask the right question concerning the traffic accidents casualties (considering the fact that the analysis is looking for the relations between the measurable features).
2. Make a graphic presentation of the distribution of the points representing the results of measuring the measurable features. Does their distribution suggest the linear character of dependence?
3. Calculate the correlation coefficient value and its significance test.
4. Did you find the directly or inversely proportional relation?
5. Estimate parameters of the (linear) regression function.
6. Mark the directional coefficient significance of the linear regression function for your example.
7. Are the marks of the linear function directional coefficient and the correlation coefficient identical? (If not, it suggests that there was a miscalculation. Why?).
8. Is it possible to discover the mechanism responsible for the dependence found?
9. Does it deserve additional data, or the answer to the question about the mechanism that causes the relation appearance can be determined upon the given data base?

# STEP 6 – exercise

# Correlation and regression

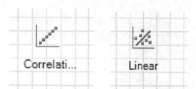

Correlati...      Linear

Analysis of the relationship between two quantitative variables aims to find a correlation coefficient and to construct a regression function. Our discussion is limited to the exploration of the linear relationship i.e. the relationship assuming a function of the form:

$$Y = A * X + B,$$

where $Y$ is a dependent variable, $X$ – an independent variable, $A$ is a slope coefficient, and $B$ denotes an intercept. Finding the A and B values identifies unequivocally the relationship between the variable $X$ and variable $Y$.

You may estimate the regression function (and at the same time the linear type of the relationship) using the available procedures as shown below.

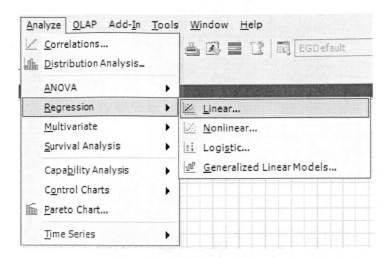

**Fig. 6.1.** Procedures associated with a regression analysis

First you define task roles (note that only quantitative variables are allowed in regression analysis):

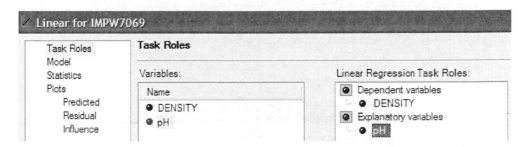

**Fig. 6.2.** Selection of variables for analysis. Drag the highlighted variable in the left window to the right window (where the arrow originally points) over an appropriate place, which at the same time defines the status of the variable, and drop

In this window you choose the appropriate option.

**Linear for IMPW5114**

Task Roles
**Model**
Statistics
Plots
   Predicted
   Residual
   Influence
Predictions
Titles

**Model**

Model selection method:

Full model fitted (no selection)

Significance levels:

To enter the model: 0.5

To stay in the model: 0.1

**Fig. 6.3.** Selection of the next option

**Linear for IMPW5114**

Task Roles
Model
Statistics
Plots
   Predicted
   Residual
   Influence
Predictions
Titles

**Statistics**

Details on estimates

☑ Standardized regression coefficients
☐ Sum of squares, Type 1
☐ Sum of squares, Type 2
☐ Correlation matrix of estimates
☐ Covariance matrix of estimates
☑ Confidence limits for parameter estimates

Confidence level: 95%

**Fig. 6.4.** Selection of parameters for calculation

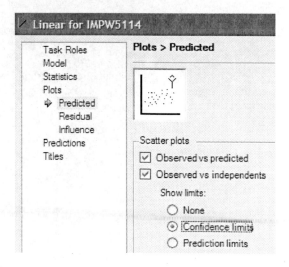

**Linear for IMPW5114**

Task Roles
Model
Statistics
Plots
 ⇨ Predicted
   Residual
   Influence
Predictions
Titles

**Plots > Predicted**

Scatter plots

☑ Observed vs predicted
☑ Observed vs independents

Show limits:

○ None
◉ Confidence limits
○ Prediction limits

**Fig. 6.5.** Selection of the graphic display

Fig. 6.6. presents graphic representation of the results (and data – results of measuring both variables) in the form of a scatter diagram with experimental points and estimated regression function. The scatter of empirical points deserves comment.

In the introduction we discussed two types of quantitative variables: continuous and stepwise variables. The pH of urine and its density are typical continuous variables (there is no numerical range that is or would be beyond the sense range). The scatter of points suggests a stepwise nature of both variables. Obviously it is a result of the accuracy of a measurement. Because of the accuracy of instruments there are numerical values on the axis that were not obtained in our study.

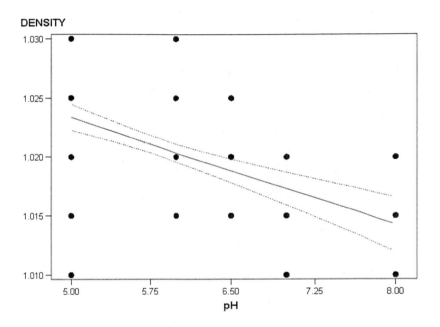

**Fig. 6.6.** Measurements (points) with the regression line and confidence intervals (the confidence limits were selected in Fig. 6.5.)

Following the selection of options (see above) i.e. confidence limits for the linear regression, two dotted lines appear on the diagram. They demarcate the area, in which there is a 95% chance that it contains the regression function after a slightly different randomization of measurements for statistical analysis. It is obvious that the area depends on the appropriate distribution of multiplicity of the data points. Although the data points are very high (for instance 1.015 for density), the confidence interval is rather narrow. It indicates the concentration of data points referring to rather low pH values over this range.

| | | | | Parameter Estimates | | | | | |
|---|---|---|---|---|---|---|---|---|---|
| Variable | Label | DF | Parameter Estimate | Standard Error | t Value | Pr > \|t\| | Standardized Estimate | 95% Confidence Limits | |
| Intercept | Intercept | 1 | 1.03852 | 0.00298 | 348.12 | <.0001 | 0 | 1.03263 | 1.04441 |
| pH | pH | 1 | -0.00303 | 0.00050813 | -5.97 | <.0001 | -0.40918 | -0.00403 | -0.00203 |

**Fig. 6.7.** Results of calculations. It appears that both the intercept and the slope coefficient of the linear regression are significantly different from zero, which means that they truly represent a set of points expressing the relationship between density and pH of urine. In the theoretical part of the book a reverse relationship is shown. Very often we do not know which variable is dependent and which is independent. You may perform calculations for both systems. You will obtain different parameter values, but their significance level will remain unaffected

If you read the table, you will find out that the regression function is of the following form in this example:

$$Density = -0.00303 * pH + 1.03852$$

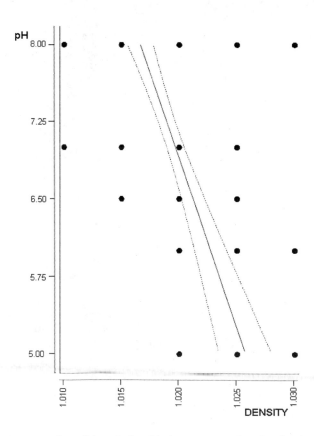

**Fig. 6.8.** Graphic representation of the relationship in a system other than in Fig. 6.6.

| Parameter Estimates | | | | | | |
|---|---|---|---|---|---|---|
| Variable | Label | DF | Parameter Estimate | Standard Error | t Value | Pr > \|t\| |
| Intercept | Intercept | 1 | 1.03852 | 0.00298 | 348.12 | <.0001 |
| pH | pH | 1 | -0.00303 | 0.00050813 | -5.97 | <.0001 |

| Parameter Estimates | | | | | | |
|---|---|---|---|---|---|---|
| Variable | Label | DF | Parameter Estimate | Standard Error | t Value | Pr > \|t\| |
| Intercept | Intercept | 1 | 62.20466 | 9.45025 | 6.58 | <.0001 |
| DENSITY | DENSITY | 1 | -55.22825 | 9.25696 | -5.97 | <.0001 |

**Fig. 6.9.** Estimation of the regression function expressing the relationship between density and pH of urine

The regression function for the relationship between density and pH of urine assumes the form:

$$pH = -55.22825 * density + 62.20466$$

Please note that the values of the linear function parameters are different. However, the character of the function is similar – it is a decreasing function in both cases (the direction of the relationship is negative).

Below you will see the next step in analysis i.e. how to determine the correlation coefficient which measures the strength of the relationship.

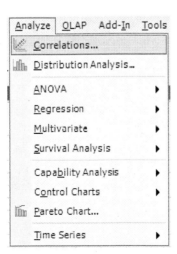

**Fig. 6.10.** Select the option to calculate the correlation coefficient

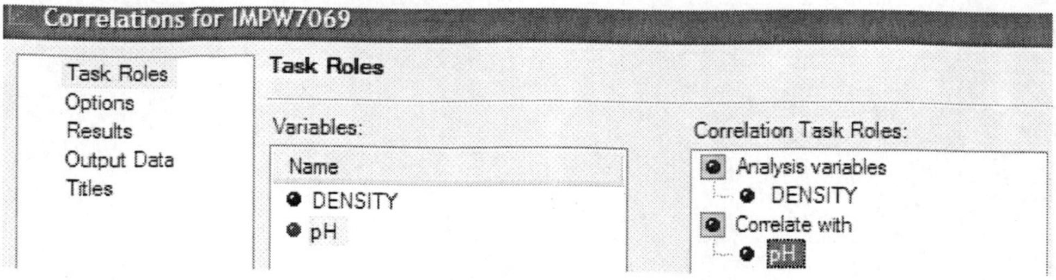

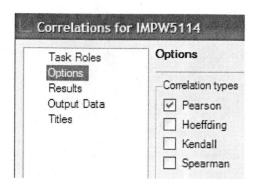

**Fig. 6.11.** Specify the task roles

**Fig. 6.12.** Select the type of the correlation coefficient (here the Pearson's correlation coefficient)

Below is the table of results:

| Simple Statistics | | | | | | | |
|---|---|---|---|---|---|---|---|
| Variable | N | Mean | Std Dev | Sum | Minimum | Maximum | Label |
| pH | 179 | 5.82402 | 0.74278 | 1043 | 5.00000 | 8.00000 | pH |
| DENSITY | 179 | 1.02087 | 0.00550 | 182.73500 | 1.01000 | 1.03000 | DENSITY |

**Fig. 6.13.** Table contains descriptive statistics describing two variables. Note that both measurements (density and pH of urine) were obtained only in 179 subjects

The correlation coefficient measuring the relationship between ph and density of urine is given in the table of results (upper line $--0.40918$) and significance level (lower line $- p < 0.0001$).

| Pearson Correlation Coefficients, N = 179 Prob > \|r\| under H0: Rho=0 | |
|---|---|
| | DENSITY |
| pH | −0.40918 |
| pH | <.0001 |

**Fig. 6.14.** Significance level of the Pearson's correlation coefficient. The p value is very low, which indicates that the obtained value differs significantly from zero, which in turn would mean no correlation between the two variables

Summing up, we demonstrated that the relationship between pH and density of urine may be described as a linear regression. Both the directional coefficient and the free variable are significant. The correlation coefficient is also significant. Both the correlation coefficient and the direction of the relationship are negative, which means that the relationship is inversely proportional. It indicates that with increasing pH of urine (decreased acidity), its density decreases.

So far the analysis has shown only that the relationship between the variables is significant. A mechanism of this relationship remains to be determined. The analysis we performed describes only the reality. Very often the role is unknown (determination of dependent and independent variables) and only specific additional studies (frequently beyond the scope of statistics) can identify the mechanism leading to the relationship we obtain.

Below is the representation of the process of calculation:

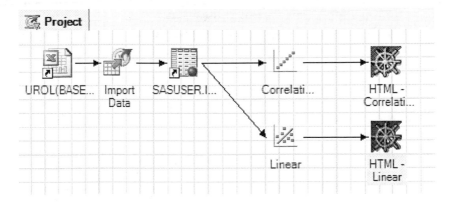

**Fig. 6.15.** Representation of the process of correlation and regression analysis

# STEP 7

## The Pearson's $\chi^2$ (chi-square) test
## (The $\chi^2$ independence test)
## Is there any relation between qualitative variables?

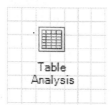

Table
Analysis

> Does the sort of diet composition influence the chemical compounds present in the stone?
> Does the accompanying illness influence the stone composition?

The diet appears to have a substantial meaning and influence upon the stone composition in the urinary tract. Several accompanying illnesses will also prove to have a connection with the stone composition in the urinary truck. The procedure called $\chi^2$ independence test will help us answer the question(s) asked.

We would like to obtain the answer expressing the mutual relation between the qualitative features. Does the kind of diet influence the stone composition? It should be noted, that the analysis is limited now only to qualitative variables. Both the diet (vegetarian, dairy, meat) and the stone composition descriptions are classic qualitative descriptions. The stone composition can be expressed only with the chemical compound name, so it is a typical qualitative variable. As it was said at the beginning, in such situations we can describe those features enumerating the number of people who belong to the given category, like the number of people with dominating vegetarian diet, etc. We can also ask about the number of people, who meet the so-called double condition, which is to say the number of people who, while preferring the vegetarian diet, have phosphates as the main component in the stone. But we are also interested in the number of people, who prefer just that type of diet and still have the oxalate salts in the stone composition. In such a situation it is the easiest to present the (numerical strength) data as a table, specifically the so-called contingency table.

The specific characteristics of such a table is determining of its size by the number of the provided form of the given feature realization forms. In our example three kinds of diet and five stone components have been differentiated. The size of our table is thus 3 × 5 (Tab. 7.1.).

| | | DIET | | | |
|---|---|---|---|---|---|
| | | MEAT | DIARY | VEGET | TOTAL |
| CHEMICAL | PHOSPHATE | 6 | 29 | 26 | 61 |
| | URIC ACID | 22 | 5 | 18 | 45 |
| | OXALATE | 36 | 12 | 96 | 144 |
| COMPOUND | CYSTINE | 1 | 2 | 1 | 4 |
| | XANTINE | 1 | 0 | 1 | 2 |
| | TOTAL | 66 | 48 | 142 | 256 |

**Tab. 7.1.** The frequencies in contingency table showing the relation of the stone composition on the patient's preferred diet

The contingency table groups the patients, placing them in appropriate cells of the table in such a way that the patient in the given cell meets both the condition of affiliation to the given column (the type of diet) and, respectively, the second condition corresponding to the affiliation to the given row (the main component of the stone). The data prepared in that way enable us to apply the test designed for finding the dependencies between the qualitative features. The test is the $\chi^2$ independence test.

Our table does not meet all the conditions that are required for the test application. The condition of applying this test is the frequency (number of observation) in each cell equal to five or higher. The xanthine and cystine stones appear very rarely. In such a situation we have two possibilities: either we cancel a given row (remove the table row from our analysis) or merge the particular rows (or columns if appropriate). The second solution is impossible in our case. The cystine stones (the stone is composed not of inorganic salts, but of amino acids, so they have nothing in common with the inorganic salts) and xanthine are of organic origin and they are difficult to combine with any other urine stone component. The combination of cystine and xanthine stones in the common category of organic provenance stones does not solve the problem, as still the number of observation in each cell would be less than five.

In order to enable performing the calculations for this issue, two rows that describe the cystine and xanthine stones get removed before the statistical test can be performed.

In order to exclude (temporarily) those people with cystine and xanthine stones, we must perform an operation of eliminating certain records from our data base, that will undergo the analysis. An example of such an operation is given in the workbook part.[41]

The final shape of the table (after excluding the people, whose main stone component is xanthine and cystine) is presented below.

| | | DIET | | | |
|---|---|---|---|---|---|
| | | MEAT | DIARY | VEGET | TOTAL |
| CHEMICAL COMPOUND | PHOSPHATE | 6 | 29 | 26 | 61 |
| | URIC ACID | 22 | 5 | 18 | 45 |
| | OXALATE | 36 | 12 | 96 | 144 |
| | TOTAL | 64 | 46 | 140 | 250 |

**Tab. 7.2.** The contingency table expressing the frequencies of he patients distribution among the categories defined in the table after the removal of CYStine and XANtine cases

In the right bottom cell, the total number of observations is given. If in any case one part of the information is lacking (the information given in rows or in columns), such a patient cannot be taken into account in our table of contingency.

The table presented in the illustration above depicts the so-called observed (experimental) frequencies.

In order to state the presence or absence of dependence between the analysed features, the observed frequencies are compared to the theoretical (expected) ones. The procedure to calculate the theoretical frequencies is organized the way to express the expected frequencies representing no dependence between variables under consideration.[42]

The theoretical frequencies are calculated on the basis of the observed frequencies.

It is the best to show the way of calculating theoretical frequencies upon an example. The expected frequencies in the cell (1,2) (row one, column two) will be obtained in the following way:

The observed frequencies sum product in row 1 and the frequencies sum product in column 2 (61*64) divided by the total number of people in the sample (250 right bottom cell) gives the expected frequency for the cell (1,2) which is 15.68. As it can be

---

[41] If we decide to combine together e.g. xantine with another compound we would have to introduce for the xantine to code common with the ingredient we would like to incorporate xantine into. For that aim we are obliged to define new variable in database. The procedure for generation the new variable is presented in workbook part.

[42] The fact has been proved mathematically, of course, which we do not present in this handbook.

seen, the theoretical frequency can (in contrast to empirical frequency) assume fraction values.

The complete table of expected (theoretical) numerical frequencies are shown in Tab. 7.3.

| | | DIET | | | |
|---|---|---|---|---|---|
| | | MEAT | DIARY | VEGET | TOTAL |
| | PHOSPHATE | 15.616 | 11.224 | 34.160 | 61 |
| CHEMICAL | URIC ACID | 11.520 | 8.280 | 25.200 | 45 |
| COMPOUND | OXALATE | 36.864 | 26.496 | 80.640 | 146 |
| | TOTAL | 64 | 46 | 140 | 258 |

**Tab. 7.3.** The expected (theoretical) frequencies for the dependence of the stone composition on the diet, calculated for empirical frequencies shown in Tab. 7.1. The theoretical numerical strength values can be expressed with the fractions (which is impossible for the empirical frequencies)

As the expected frequencies express a complete absence of dependencies, it is obvious, that the higher the difference between them and the observed ones, the stronger is the dependence between two variables under consideration. The discussed test statistics value is expressed as the difference value (for all the cells in the table) between the theoretical (expected) and the observed frequency in the relative scale (the components divided by the adequate theoretical frequency).

A detailed testing procedure according to $\chi^2$ *independence test* (Pearson's $\chi^2$ test) is given below:

1. Hypothesis:

   $H_0$ – the frequency distribution observed in a sample is consistent with a particular theoretical distribution (there are no dependencies between the analysed qualitative features).
   $H_1$ – the frequency distribution observed in a sample is inconsistent with a particular theoretical distribution (there is a dependence between the analysed qualitative features).

2. The objectiveness conditions:

   A – the number of degrees of freedom $df = (r-1)*(s-1)$,              (eq. 7.1.)

   $r$ – signifies the number of columns in the table (excluding the collective column),
   $s$ – the number of rows (excluding the row of sums).
   B – the significance level – assumed ($\alpha = 5\%$).

3. The statistics value (the quantitative evaluation criterion):

$$\chi^2 = \sum_{i=1}^{r} \sum_{j=1}^{s} \frac{(n_{ij} - np_{ij})^2}{np_{ij}}$$ (eq. 7.2.)

or equivalent

$$\chi^2 = n \sum_{i=1}^{r} \frac{(p_{ti} - p_{ei})^2}{p_{ti}}$$ (eq. 7.3.)

4. The critical value read from the tables for the given number of degrees of freedom and the

given significance level $\chi^2_{crit.}(df, \alpha)$ – the critical area.
Or the read *"p"* value for the appointed statistics value (point 3).

5. The final decision:
$p < \alpha$ – $H_0$ is rejected.
$p > \alpha$ – there are no grounds for $H_0$ rejection.

Or:

$\chi^2_{calc.} < \chi^2_{crit.}(df, \alpha)$ – there is no reason for $H_0$ rejection

$\chi^2_{calc.} > \chi^2_{crit.}(df, \alpha)$ – $H_0$ is rejected.

6. Interpretation of final results.

## INTERPRETATION

If $H_0$ of $\chi^2$ *independence test* is rejected, we state that the dependence between the diet and the main stone component is present and that this dependency is quite strong. In our case it signifies that the diet influences the stone component in the urinary system (see the results in workbook). However, this is not ultimately satisfying for us. We would also like to learn or explain the mechanism responsible of such dependence. In order to obtain the answer to the question about the source of such dependence we can do another test, which will help us to identify the mechanism that leads to such dependence or suggest an additional (biochemical) analytical experimental examination. The wanted mechanism can assume any of the forms already presented when discussing looking for dependence between the measurable features.

Coming back again to looking for the relations between the qualitative features, let us check if the presence of an accompanying illness, which is for example cardiac disease, has anything in common with the main stone component.
The table below (already after the removal of a small group of those people in whom cystine or xanthine) shows the empirical frequencies in the contingency table cells (rows – two – distinguish the patients with and without circulation system disease).

The columns (as in the previous example) identify the dominating component of the deposit.

The test result is shown in the table 7.4.

| | | HART DISEASE | | | |
|---|---|---|---|---|---|
| | | YES | NO | TOTAL | DECISION |
| CHEMICAL COMPOUND | PHOSPHATE | 9 | 52 | 61 | $p = 0.925$ No dependence |
| | URIC ACID | 11 | 32 | 43 | |
| | OXALATE | 27 | 119 | 146 | |
| | TOTAL | 47 | 203 | 250 | |

**Tab. 7.4.** The table of empirical frequencies showing the relation of the presence of heart disease appearance in connection with the stone composition. In the right column the results of the conducted test were presented, indicating the absence of any relation between these features

As we can see, there is no relation between the presence of cardiac disease and the stone composition. Heart diseases do not influence the composition of organic fluids that can cause the stone appearance in the urinary tract.

Both quoted examples show, that the $\chi^2$ *independence test* analyses the contingency table regardless of its size. The smallest table size is $2 \times 2$. The only limitation for this test is the frequency in each cell of the table, which must be higher than 5.

# Exercises

1. Ask a question concerning finding the relation between the qualitative features describing the traffic accidents casualties.
2. What is the contingency table size?
3. Are the frequencies in all cells higher than 4?
4. What solution can be chosen to avoid the problem of low frequency? Removing row (or column) or rather joining of particular categories is appropriate to solve this problem?
5. Does the significant relation found between the qualitative features need further analyses in order to assign the mechanism responsible for the relations appearance?

# STEP 7 – exercise

# $\chi^2$ (chi-square) test of independence

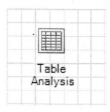

Analysis of qualitative variables is based mainly on numbers of elements (patients) fulfilling the criteria defined for a given table of contingency. Click the "**Describe**" drop-down menu on the main menu bar and select "**Table Analysis**".

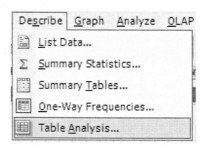

**Fig. 7.1.** Select the Table Analysis option to investigate the relationship between the qualitative variables

As usual, you have to define variable roles to analyze.

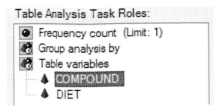

**Fig. 7.2.** Define the role of a variable. Both variables are qualitative

Place the cursor on the selected variable, press down the left mouse button, drag the variable and drop it in the right column or row.

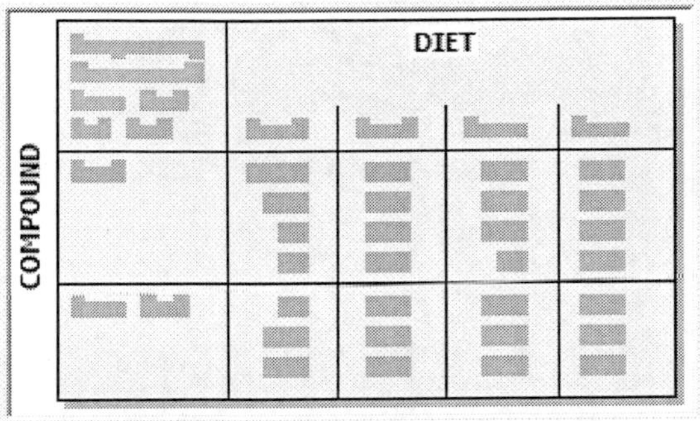

**Fig. 7.3.** Contingency table constructed of data in appropriate columns and rows

In the second step you define which information you expect to obtain as a description of cells in the contingency table.

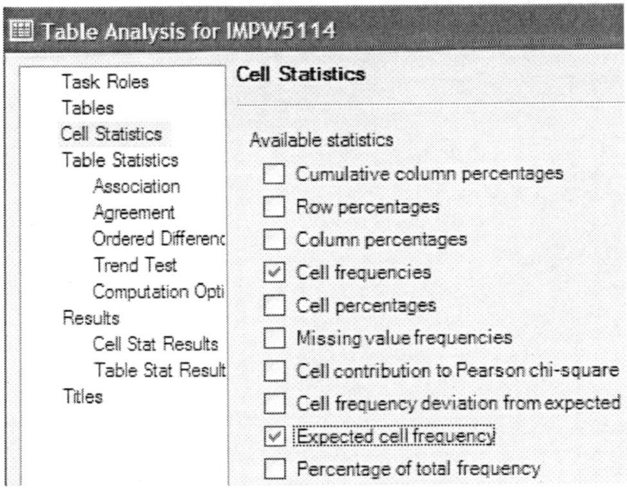

**Fig. 7.4.** Select the parameters you want to obtain in a result set. Table of results will contain the observed and expected data

You have selected the observed and expected cell frequencies.

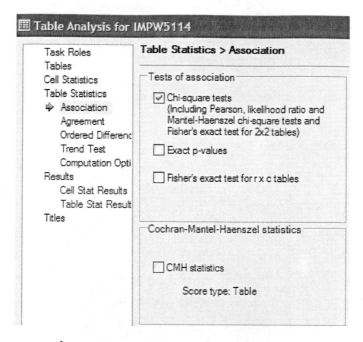

**Fig. 7.5.** You expect a $\chi^2$ test will be performed

You select the test you plan to perform using the contingency table in order to investigate the relationship between the variables (COMPOUND and DIET).

| Frequency Expected | Table of DIET by COMPOUND | | | | | |
|---|---|---|---|---|---|---|
| | COMPOUND(COMPOUND) | | | | | |
| DIET(DIET) | CYS | XANT | OXALATE | PHOSPHATE | URICAC | Total |
| MEAT | 0 0.5403 | 1 0.2702 | 24 32.419 | 6 13.778 | 36 19.992 | 67 |
| MILK | 2 0.3871 | 0 0.1935 | 11 23.226 | 29 9.871 | 6 14.323 | 48 |
| VEGET | 0 1.0726 | 0 0.5363 | 85 64.355 | 16 27.351 | 32 39.685 | 133 |
| Total | 2 | 1 | 120 | 51 | 74 | 248 |

Frequency Missing = 6

**Fig. 7.6.** Table (as defined in Fig. 7.4.) provides observed data (upper row) and theoretical data (lower row). There are cells with very small data (below 5)

As you may see there are two values in the cells. The upper value is the observed frequency and the lower value the theoretical one.

Below is the table, which contains also the results of other tests apart from the $\chi^2$ test. A brief comment in the bottom of the table is important. You are informed that the results of the test may be unreliable because of too small values in the cells. In this situation you may merge some columns (or rows), but only when it is justifiable from the viewpoint of analysis (you cannot merge cells if it is not reasonable). Another option would be to skip small samples.

| Statistic | DF | Value | Prob |
|---|---|---|---|
| Chi-Square | 8 | 91.5945 | <.0001 |
| Likelihood Ratio Chi-Square | 8 | 79.1175 | <.0001 |
| Mantel-Haenszel Chi-Square | 1 | 15.6760 | <.0001 |
| Phi Coefficient | | 0.6077 | |
| Contingency Coefficient | | 0.5193 | |
| Cramer's V | | 0.4297 | |
| WARNING: 40% of the cells have expected counts less than 5. Chi-Square may not be a valid test. | | | |

Fig. 7.7. Table of results. All tests (you selected only the $\chi^2$ test) indicate that the relationship between the variables is significant

In this example because of too small samples of patients with cystine and xanthine stones, we decided to exclude these two types of stones from analysis.

| Frequency Expected | Table of DIET by COMPOUND | | | |
|---|---|---|---|---|
| | COMPOUND(COMPOUND) | | | |
| DIET(DIET) | OXALATE | PHOSPHATE | URICAC | Total |
| MEAT | 24<br>32.327 | 6<br>13.739 | 36<br>19.935 | 66 |
| MILK | 11<br>22.531 | 29<br>9.5755 | 6<br>13.894 | 46 |
| VEGET | 85<br>65.143 | 16<br>27.686 | 32<br>40.171 | 133 |
| Total | 120 | 51 | 74 | 245 |

**Fig. 7.8.** Contingency table (the observed and expected frequencies) after skipping small samples (CYS and XANT)

Above is the same table after skipping small samples.

| Frequency Row Pct Col Pct | Table of DIET by COMPOUND | | | |
|---|---|---|---|---|
| | COMPOUND(COMPOUND) | | | |
| DIET(DIET) | OXALATE | PHOSPHATE | URICAC | Total |
| MEAT | 24<br>36.36<br>20.00 | 6<br>9.09<br>11.76 | 36<br>54.55<br>48.65 | 66 |
| MILK | 11<br>23.91<br>9.17 | 29<br>63.04<br>56.86 | 6<br>13.04<br>8.11 | 46 |
| VEGET | 85<br>63.91<br>70.83 | 16<br>12.03<br>31.37 | 32<br>24.06<br>43.24 | 133 |
| Total | 120 | 51 | 74 | 245 |

**Fig. 7.9.** Output of the table shows the number of occurrences in each cell and the percentage this represents of the column and row

This time each cell contains the number of observed occurrences and the percentage this represents of the row and column (calculated for a given stone constituent and type of diet).

*Statistics for Table of DIET by COMPOUND*

| Statistic | DF | Value | Prob |
|---|---|---|---|
| Chi-Square | 4 | 81.8880 | <.0001 |
| Likelihood Ratio Chi-Square | 4 | 69.8680 | <.0001 |
| Mantel-Haenszel Chi-Square | 1 | 20.0199 | <.0001 |
| Phi Coefficient | | 0.5781 | |
| Contingency Coefficient | | 0.5005 | |
| Cramer's V | | 0.4088 | |

**Fig. 7.10.** Results of the test show that the relationship between the variables (stone component and diet) is significant

This table contains the results of the tests (no comment this time), indicating that $H_0$ should be rejected. It means that the type of diet has a significant impact on the main component of renal stones. This fact may be easily interpreted. Nutrients in the foods we eat are dissolved in the blood and when the concentration of certain salts in urine (especially when the diet is monotonous) exceeds the limits of solubility, the salts crystallize and form stones within the kidneys.

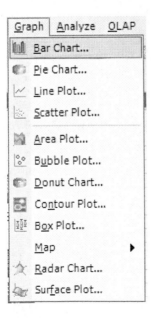

**Fig. 7.11.** List graphic display options

178

You may choose the form of graphic display from the Bar Chart menu.

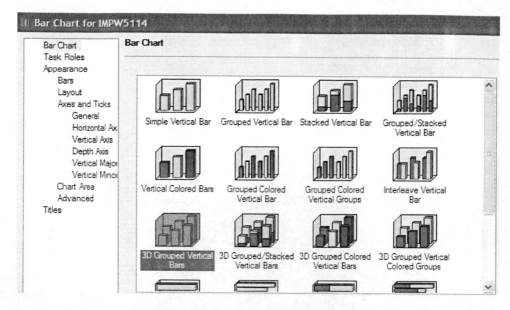

**Fig. 7.12.** List of bar charts with 3D grouped vertical bars are highlighted

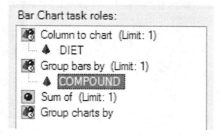

**Fig. 7.13.** Define the variables you want to display in the graphic form

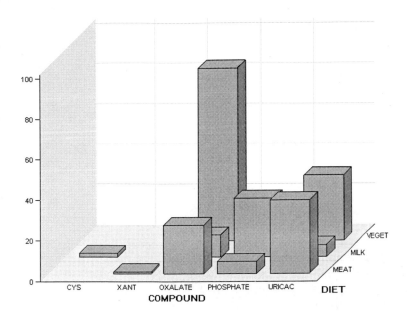

**Fig. 7.14.** Bars representing all groups (including small samples)

Above is a graphic display of the results before skipping small samples and excluding the records with missing data.

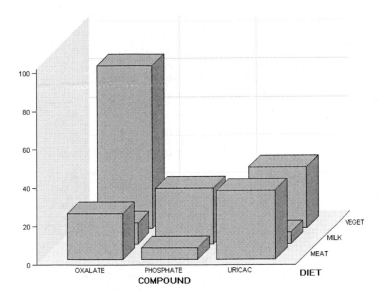

**Fig. 7.15.** The same bar chart after skipping small samples

Fig. 7.15. displays the number of subjects in groups divided by dominating diet and stone component.

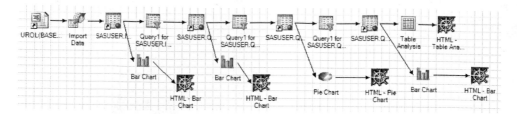

**Fig. 7.16.** Representation of the process of analysis

Fig. 7.16. is to remind you the process of analysis. The primary database was modified three times (Query), filtered to exclude records with missing data (if one variable is not defined, the record must be excluded from analysis) and then data referring to cystine and xanthine stones.

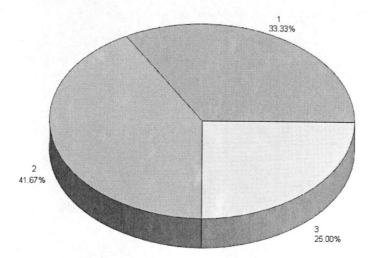

**Fig. 7.17.** Pie chart showing proportions of diet in our study group

In another form of graphic display, pie chart shows proportions of individuals on various types of diet (Fig. 7.17.).

In this example the $\chi^2$ test was used to show the significant relationship between two variables – diet and stone composition.
Identical calculations can be performed for other variables i.e. blood and bacteria in urine and the results are shown below.

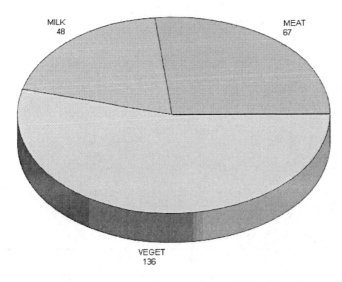

**Pie Chart**

MILK
48

MEAT
67

VEGET
136

| Frequency Expected | Table of BLOOD by BACTERIA | | | |
|---|---|---|---|---|
| | | BACTERIA(BACTERIA) | | |
| BLOOD(BLOOD) | | N | Y | Total |
| N | | 17 17.246 | 38 37.754 | 55 |
| Y | | 57 56.754 | 124 124.25 | 181 |
| Total | | 74 | 162 | 236 |

**Fig. 7.18.** Contingency table to investigate the relationship between blood and bacteria in urine

*Statistics for Table of BLOOD by BACTERIA*

| Statistic | DF | Value | Prob |
|---|---|---|---|
| Chi-Square | 1 | 0.0067 | 0.9350 |
| Likelihood Ratio Chi-Square | 1 | 0.0067 | 0.9349 |
| Continuity Adj. Chi-Square | 1 | 0.0000 | 1.0000 |
| Mantel-Haenszel Chi-Square | 1 | 0.0066 | 0.9351 |
| Phi Coefficient | | -0.0053 | |
| Contingency Coefficient | | 0.0053 | |
| Cramer's V | | -0.0053 | |

**Fig. 7.19.** Table of results investigating the relationship between blood and bacteria in urine. You should accept $H_0$, which indicates no relationship between these two variables

In this example there is no relationship between blood and bacteria in urine. It means that the presence of blood in urine is caused by a different reason.

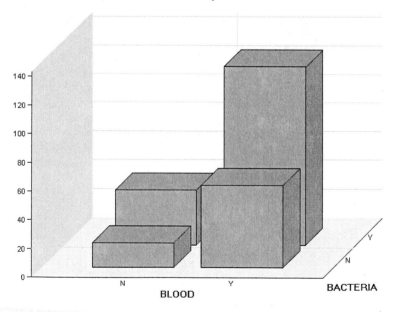

**Fig. 7.20.** Graphic display for contingency table investigating the relationship between blood (present Y, absent N) and bacteria in urine (present Y and absent N)

Fig. 7.20. a graphic presentation of the results investigating the relationship between blood and bacteria in urine.

# STEP 8

# Nonparametric tests (distribution-free tests) How about the data not representing the normal distribution?

Nonparame...
One-Way A...

> Does the age of female patients with nephrolithiasis urinary tract nephrolithiasis differ from the age of male patients with the same illness?
> Is the urine pH in the patients with bacteriuria different in relation to the patients without the urinary tract infection?
> Does the urine pH really specifically differ in groups created according to the stone localization?
> Does the stone localization determine the patient's body temperature?
> Is the patient's age really different for the groups with a different accompanying illness?

At the very beginning of the course we stated that the women's age did not represent the normal distribution. We could not make use of the already familiar T-test comparing the two arithmetic mean values, as the women's age mean could not be treated as a parameter of normal distribution, and only in such a situation the T-test is applied. The age comparison is possible, though with the application of nonparametric tests, which can be applied for the values that not necessarily represent the normal distribution.

In order to answer the questions asked, we should return to the scheme in Fig. 5.2. If it proves that the measurable feature distribution in any distinctive (compared) group does not represent the normal distribution in the light of the test checking the distribution type, one should refer to the nonparametric tests. The age in women patients group has a distribution different from normal. So if we want to know the answer, if there is a statistically significant difference between the age of men and women reporting to hospital because of nephrolithiasis, it is only now when we refer to the nonparametric tests, that we can answer that question.

As the name itself indicates, those are the tests that do not refer to any type of distribution, and they do not require any initial assumptions or conditioning.

We compare the age (the measurable feature of the distribution different from normal) in two groups (men and women).

What does the analysis technique like in such a case? The nonparametric tests are based on ranking procedure. Instead of defining this procedure theoretically, let us refer to an example.

We arrange the number of the patients' years in a common series, although we mark the group from which the given result comes from. A sample series (fragmentary) was shown below.

| 21 32 81 54 56 47 32 41 58 71 62 | 64 69 53 53 62 19 36 51 68 53 57 73 47 67 39 41 48 46 |
|---|---|

19 21 32 32 36 39 41 41 46 47 47   48 51 53 53 53 54 56 57 58 62 62 64 67 68 69 71 73 81

1 2 3 4 5 6 7 8 9 10 11 12 13 14 15 16 17 18 19 20 21 22 23 24 25 26 27 28 29

1 2 3.5 3.5 5 6 7.5 7.5 9 10.5 10.5 12 13 15 15 15 17 18 19 20 21.5 21.5 23 24 25 26 27 28 29

| 2 3.5 3.5 7.5 10.5 17 18 20 21.5 27 29 | 1 5 6 7.5 9 10.5 12 13 15 15 15 19 21.5 23 24 25 26 28 |
|---|---|
| 159.5 | 275.5 |
| 11 | 18 |

19 21 32 32 36 39 41 41 46 47 47   48 51 53 53 53 54 56 57 58 62 62 64 67 68 69 71 73 81

⇑

|  | GROUP A | GROUP B | TOTAL |
|---|---|---|---|
| =<Me | 5 | 11 | 16 |
| >Me | 6 | 7 | 13 |
| TOTAL | 11 | 18 | 29 |

**Tab. 8.1.** The steps in ranking procedure

The 1-st row – left site represents the age of women (F) in the chronological order (as appeared in database), the right site – the age of men (M) in chronological order. The values related to women are given in bold in this table.

The 2-nd row – the number of years put together (F + M) in increasing order. The bold numbers represent F.

The 3-th – the values of ranks are attached to each age value – pay attention on those ages, which appeared in more than once.

The 4-th row – the brackets distinguishing the repeated values.

The 5-th row – the ranks values calculated as averaged values for positions of equal values.

The 6-th row – the F and M ranks values separated according to the gender

The 7-th row – sum of ranks for each gender-group

The 8-ht row – number of elements in each group

The 9-th row – the arrow points the position of median

The table (contingency table) represents the numbers belonging to classes generated versus the Me value (which has been found to be equal to 53)

The Wilcoxon test takes the lower rank sum value as the value of statistics

The Kruskal-Wallis test takes the sum of ranks (and number of elements in each group)

The median test – performance as in $\chi^2$ test (independence) according to the contingency table generated in relation to the Me value for the common set of data.


The gender differentiation (women) were marked with bold print. The position of each value in the series is numbered (row 2). The number in the position in the ordered series signifies the so-called rank. As it can be seen, several age positions assume the same values. Two identical values of a measured feature cannot have two different positions ascribed. Then two (or more) equal values assume the rank value equal to the arithmetic mean of those primary values. It has been shown in the setting-up account (row 3).

In the next step we come back to the initial division into two groups, keeping the rank of each value in the series.

In the last step, we separately calculate ranks sum of all the elements that belong to each group separately.

The data so prepared can be then analysed with the help of a statistical test based upon the ranking procedure.

It is obvious to comment, that a large discrepancy between the sums of ranks calculated for the separate groups suggests, that the elements coming from one group were concentrated round the low ranks, while the high sum of ranks in the second group suggests, that in this group the ranked values were placed in the final part of the common ordered series. As it can be seen, no data-describing parameter is needed in the ranking procedure. This is why these tests are called also distribution-free tests. The sum of ranks value (or values) is (are) estimated in nonparametric tests.

We refer to the already known testing procedure, this time presenting the test of Wilcoxon:

1. $H_0$ – There are no differences between the compared groups.

   It should be noted that we are not comparing any specific parameter or any value. We make a general statement about the groups similarity without specifying any parameter.

   Another $H_0$ of this test sounds: both samples come from the same population, which signifies, that there is no factor that would differentiate those two groups.

   $H_1$ – the samples come from different populations.

2. The objectivity parameters:

   A – the number of degrees of freedom

   $$df = n_{min} \qquad \text{(eq. 8.1.)}$$

   The number of degrees of freedom is equal to the size value of the sample with a lower number of elements

   B – the significance level – assumed 5%.

3. The statistics value is just equal to the sum of ranks for the group of lower number of elements:

   $$R_{n,min} \qquad \text{(eq. 8.2.)}$$

4. The critical value (read from tables or calculated by the programme):
   Or the "p" value corresponding to the calculated statistics value (calculated by the programme).

5. If $p > \alpha$ – there are no grounds for rejecting $H_0$.
   If $p > \alpha$ – $H_0$ is rejected.

6. Interpretation.

The result of the test made in order to compare the male and female patients' age with urine tract nephrolithiasis shows that, from the point of view of this feature, the illness appears in the comparable period of life (see the workbook part).

If we assume, that the distribution of pH in the group of patients with haematuria differed from normal, the only possibility would be comparing the urine acidity in the two groups exactly on the basis of Wilcoxon test.

Another example of a nonparametric test is the Wilcoxon-Mann-Whitney test.

Like the Wilcoxon test presented above, it also compares two groups. The only difference with respect to Wilcoxon test is the way of calculating the statistics value (although it is based on the rank values).

1. $H_0$ – there are no differences between the compared groups.

It should be noted that we are not comparing any specific parameter or any value. We make a general statement of the groups similarity without specifying any parameter.

Another form of this test's $H_0$ sounds: both samples come from the same population, so there is no factor that would differentiate these two groups.

$H_1$ – each sample comes from a different population.

2. The objective parameters:

A – the number of degrees of freedom

$$df_1 = n \text{ number of elements in the group of lower size} \qquad \text{(eq. 8.3.)}$$

B – the significance level – assumed 5%.

3. The statistics value:

$$U = nm + \frac{n(n+1)}{2} - R_1 \qquad \text{(eq. 8.4.)}$$

where: $n$ – number of elements in lower size group
$m$ – number of elements in higher size group,
$Rn$ – sum of the ranks in the group of lower number of elements in the group

4. The critical value of statistics or *"p"* value :

IF $p < \alpha$ – $H_0$ is rejected.
IF $p > \alpha$ – there are no grounds to reject $H_0$.

5. Decision.

6. Interpretation.

If there is a necessity to compare a larger number of groups of people, among which at least one's distribution is different from normal, we refer to Kruskal-Wallis test, considered as nonparametric ANOVA equivalent. We refer to this test in order to find the answer to the question concerning the relation between the patient's age and his/her professional activity. We are going to compare the patients' age in five groups, as five professions have been provided.

The result table set is presented in the workbook part.

Here we remind the stages of testing using the test described:

1. $H_0$ – there are no differences between the groups compared. It should be noted, that we do not compare any specific parameter or any value. We make a general statement concerning the group similarity without specifying any parameter.

    Another $H_0$ form of this test is: all samples come from the same population, so there is no factor to differentiate these groups.

    $H_1$ – each sample comes from a different population.

2. The objectivity parameters:

    A – the number of degrees of freedom

    $df = k - 1$     where $k$ – number of compared groups          (eq. 8.5.)

    B – the significance level – assumed – 5%.

3. The statistics value:

$$H = \frac{12}{n(n+1)} \sum_{i=1}^{k} \frac{T_i^2}{n_i} - 3(n+1)$$          (eq. 8.6.)

where: $n$ – (total number of elements) $= \sum_{i=1}^{k} n_i$ ,

$n_i$ – size of the sample (number of elements),
$T_i$ – sum of ranks in a given group,
$k$ – number of groups.

4. The critical value from the tables

    The "$p$" value

5. The final decision:

    IF $p < \alpha$ – $H_0$ is rejected
    IF $p > \alpha$ – there is no reason to reject $H_0$

6. Interpretation.

An example of a test that combines the elements of the ranking procedure and contingency table construction is the test of median.
In this example, the following question will be asked:
Does long immobilization influence the age of nephrolithiasis appearance?
According to the questionnaire (Tab. 1. STEP 1) we differentiated two groups: people chronically immobilized (patients with MS, accident casualties) and the people free to move. A jointly created series allows us for the specification of the number of people who represent the age above the median and below it. As a result we obtain the contingency table (exactly such as the one that we analysed in the case of $\chi^2$ independence test) and perform the $\chi^2$ independence test. The difference consists only in the fact that

the division into the age categories is evaluated in relation to the values of median in a common ordered series (in our case it is a series of ordered values specifying the patient's age).

An operation of dividing the people into two groups assuming the median values as the division criterion, can be an example of changing the measurable feature status, i.e. the age, to the qualitative feature status, as we estimate the patient's age only as below or above the median value.

The result obtained (the exercises part) suggests, that long immobilization influences the deposit appearance. We found that the age of immobilized patients is substantially lower (the comparison of rank values sum) than the age of nephrolithiasis appearance in the mobile patients.

It is extremely difficult to present the partial results (each step of procedure) due to the operation of large number of values. It is assumed, that the Reader knowing the procedures of other statistical tests understands the operation performed by the computer. Although the procedures applied in all tests presented in this STEP 8 are shown in Tab. 8.1.

# Summarizing information

There are several subjects to be covered in order to learn the statistics basics that have been gathered in this chapter, which are:
1. Estimation of the confidence interval for the normal distribution parameters, and
2. Estimation of the minimum size for the sample, in order to treat it as representative.

## The confidence interval once again

As it has already been told, we do not know the value of the arithmetic mean describing the population. In such uncertainty conditions, appreciated information is specifying the range interval in which an unknown arithmetic mean with a definite probability can appear.

The area is specified with the name of confidence interval.

We have already told that the area specified with the formula:

$$\bar{x} - 1.96\sigma < x < \bar{x} + 1.96\sigma \qquad \text{(eq. 8.7.)}$$

gives the range, in which we are going to find the values x with the probability of 95%.

Obviously, the same formula for the sample parameters has the following form:

$$\bar{x} - 1.96s < x < \bar{x} + 1.96s \qquad \text{(eq. 8.8.)}$$

We know that each calculated value of the arithmetic mean bears an error. We also know that drawing another sample can produce (and it does) another parameter value, which is the arithmetic mean. In such a situation statistics refers to the procedure of drawing multiple samples, for which the values of the arithmetic mean are calculated. After the procedure multiple repetition and multiple calculation of the arithmetic mean values for each draw it will prove, that the distribution of the mean values has also a strictly defined form compliant with the distribution of the T-Student test, which is described (variable $t$ analogous to variable $Z$) by the following formula:

$$t = \frac{\bar{x} - m}{s/\sqrt{n}} \qquad \text{(eq. 8.9.)}$$

So, if we are looking for the confidence interval for the value of the arithmetic mean from the sample, the confidence interval is then calculated with the following formula:

$$P\left\{ \bar{x} - t_{\alpha/2, n-1} \cdot \frac{s}{\sqrt{n-1}} < m < \bar{x} + t_{\alpha/2, n-1} \cdot \frac{s}{\sqrt{n-1}} \right\} = 1 - \alpha, \qquad \text{(eq. 8.10.)}$$

where: $P$ – signifies the probability for the confidence interval in the above example it is 95% (because it was defined as $1 - \alpha$, where $\alpha$ signifies the assumed significance level, which is to say 5%); $\bar{x}$ – signifies our calculated arithmetic mean (from the sample); $s$ – signifies the value of standard deviation (for the sample); $m$ – expresses that unknown mean that fits into the assigned interval with the assumed $P$; the symbols $t_{\alpha/2, n-1}$ – signify the statistics value for the t-Student distribution for the assumed level of $\alpha$ and the number of degrees of freedom $= n - 1$.[43]

The statistical packets give also the confidence intervals for the remaining parameters of normal distribution, i.e. for the variance and the standard deviation.

**The minimum size for the representative sample**
**The representative sample**

As it has already been said, the objective of statistical analysis is the population description on the basis of sample testing. Such generalization is only possible at a large enough size of the sample.

Appointing the minimum size for the representative sample is based upon the results of the so-called pilot sample, which need not be representative.

The minimum size for the sample, which can be treated as representative, can be calculated using the following formula (with an assumption of the confidence level and a margin of the estimation error):

$$n = \frac{t_{\alpha}^2 \hat{s}^2}{d^2},$$ 
(eq. 8.11.)

where: $n$ – signifies the required size of the representative sample; $t_{\alpha}^2$ – expresses the square of values $t$ for the significance level (confidence interval) $\alpha$; $\hat{s}^2$ – signifies the variance calculated for the pilot sample value; and $d$ – signifies the maximum acceptable, assumed in advance estimation value of the mean (the value expressed in the measurement units).

# Exercises

1. Ask a question concerning the traffic accidents casualties, for which the answer will be obtained upon the median test.
2. Perform the median test
3. Have you found the median value for the measurable feature present in the above example?

---

[43] The formula given above can be individually derived. The inquisitive Readers are suggested to conduct such a transformation. There remains an unknown expression $\alpha/2$. We leave this expression explanation to the inquisitive Readers, too. We can prompt, that it is connected with the notion of one- and two-sided test.

4. Make the test of Kruskal-Wallis with respect to the appropriate data (features) present in the data base concerning the traffic accidents casualties, on the basis of the example placed in this chapter.

5. Have you done a prior analysis in order to specify the distribution type of the measurable feature?

# STEP 8 – exercise

# Nonparametric tests (distribution free tests)

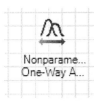

Nonparame...
One-Way A...

We stated before that the distribution of ages among females is not normal. For this reason we could not characterize the distribution of ages among males as compared with females.

In this situation we use nonparametric tests. Analysis dialog boxes have already been presented, so this time you can see the final results.

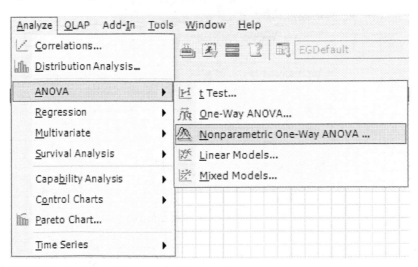

**Fig. 8.1.** Dialog box to select a nonparametric procedure

Below is a table summarizing values for the Wilcoxon rank sum test.

| Wilcoxon Scores (Rank Sums) for Variable AGE Classified by Variable GENDER | | | | | |
|---|---|---|---|---|---|
| GENDER | N | Sum of Scores | Expected Under H0 | Std Dev Under H0 | Mean Score |
| M | 158 | 18340.50 | 19908.0 | 555.351451 | 116.079114 |
| F | 93 | 13285.50 | 11718.0 | 555.351451 | 142.854839 |
| Average scores were used for ties. | | | | | |

**Fig. 8.2.** Table comparing age of women and men with urolithiasis

Test results and p value to state similarities or differences in age distribution between men and women are given below.

| Wilcoxon Two-Sample Test | |
|---|---|
| Statistic | 13285.5000 |
| | |
| Normal Approximation | |
| Z | 2.8216 |
| One-Sided Pr > Z | 0.0024 |
| Two-Sided Pr > \|Z\| | 0.0048 |
| | |
| t Approximation | |
| One-Sided Pr > Z | 0.0026 |
| Two-Sided Pr > \|Z\| | 0.0052 |

**Fig. 8.3.** Test results showing a significant difference in age between women and men (very low p values in all tests)

As shown, p values in all tests are below 5%. It means that the null hypothesis that there is no difference between the two samples should be rejected. It further means that from the viewpoint of age women with urolithiasis differ from men with urolithiasis. It serves as a starting point for search for other causes of such differences.

| Kruskal-Wallis Test | |
|---|---|
| Chi-Square | 7.9667 |
| DF | 1 |
| Pr > Chi-Square | 0.0048 |

**Fig. 8.4.** Result of the Kruskal-Wallis test indicating a significant difference in age between females and males

The Kruskal-Wallis test result is also near zero, which means that the null hypothesis that there is no difference in age between women and men should be rejected.

| Median Scores (Number of Points Above Median) for Variable AGE Classified by Variable GENDER | | | | | |
|---|---|---|---|---|---|
| GENDER | N | Sum of Scores | Expected Under H0 | Std Dev Under H0 | Mean Score |
| M | 158 | 70.50 | 78.685259 | 3.771662 | 0.446203 |
| F | 93 | 54.50 | 46.314741 | 3.771662 | 0.586022 |
| Average scores were used for ties. | | | | | |

**Fig. 8.5.** Results of the median test

The median test selected in the dialog box defining the test criteria also shows that the null hypothesis should be rejected.

| Median Two-Sample Test | |
|---|---|
| Statistic | 54.5000 |
| Z | 2.1702 |
| One-Sided Pr > Z | 0.0150 |
| Two-Sided Pr > |Z| | 0.0300 |

**Fig. 8.6.** Final results of the median test indicate a significant difference in age between men and women with urolithiasis

| Median One-Way Analysis | |
|---|---|
| Chi-Square | 4.7098 |
| DF | 1 |
| Pr > Chi-Square | 0.0300 |

**Fig. 8.7.** Another type of median test (as mentioned before SAS package offers a lot more than its users expect) also indicates a significant difference

We found out that age of women and men is derived from two unequal populations. What is the factor that differentiates the distribution of ages among women and men with urolithiasis?

# STEP 9

# COMPREHENSIVE ANALYSIS

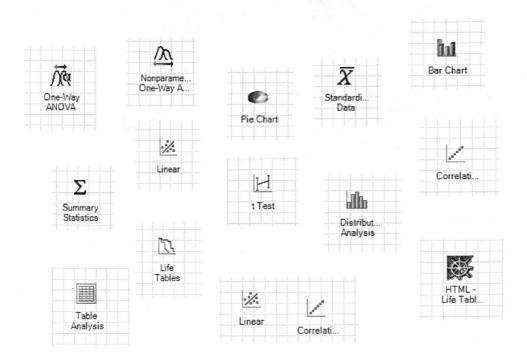

## | Do we know already the method to prevent nephrolithiasis?

At the beginning of our discussion we posed a question that we would like to solve by means of the statistical analysis method. In order to present the particular tests we asked particular questions. By now, neither of the tests has produced an answer if, and to what extent we can prevent the appearance of stone deposit appearance in the urinary tract area. This question will be answered after performing a series of tests properly suited to the particular data issues.

An analysis of the medical problem requires using numerous tests that provide answers to closely specified questions. Setting the given answers and their complex analysis will let us find the ways of nephrolithiasis prevention.

## Is the anatomical defect of the urinary system influencing the nephrolithiasis?

We have already said that the presence of congenital defect in a given person results as earlier nephrolithiasis appearance in comparison with those patients where the defect is absent. Two groups, obtained in relation to the information concerning the family interview, (nephrolithiasis presence in the family YES/NO question, (see a questionnaire STEP 1)) were compared from the point of view of patients' age. It should be checked if the distribution of age in both groups is the normal distribution. If so, (this was checked and the $\chi^2$ accordance test confirmed the presence of normal distribution in both groups), the t-Student test can be performed. The results are given below.

| CONGENITAL DEFECTS | AGE (years) | | | TEST applied | p | $H_0$ | DECISION |
|---|---|---|---|---|---|---|---|
| | n | $\bar{x}$ | s | | | | |
| ABSENT | 205 | 51.9 | 13.7 | F | 0.47 | No rejection | Dispersion – no differences |
| PRESENT | 51 | 34.7 | 14.6 | t | 0.0001 | REJECT | Mean values – difference significant |

**Tab. 9.1.** The table presents the descriptive characteristics of the variable – age in two groups (with and without congenital defects) and the results of applying two tests: F – comparing the dispersions of age in both groups which appeared to be not different and t-Student test which compares the averaged age between these two groups. It was shown that the average age is significantly different in compared groups[44]

---

[44] This is the good example for one- and two-sided test to be applied. Two-sided test ($H_1$ – difference is significant $m_{with} \neq m_{without}$) states that the difference is significant. The one-side test ($H_1$ – the averaged age in the second group significantly higher than in the first one $m_{with} < m_{without}$) points out the group of higher risk to get nephrolithiasis.

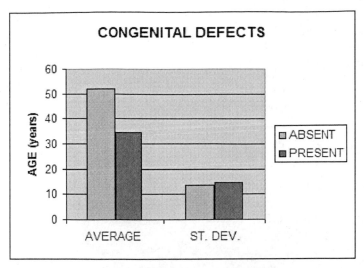

**Fig. 9.1.** The graphic presentation of parameters describing the age in group of patients with and without congenital defects (mean values and standard deviations respectively)

**Interpretation**
There is a difference between the patients' age **with** the congenital defect and **without** the congenital defect found. Renal nephrolithiasis appears significantly earlier in the (considerably younger) people with the anatomical defect

The interpretation causes the conclusion that in case of a positive family interview nephrolithiasis can be supposed at a substantially earlier age in comparison to those people in whose families nephrolithiasis has not appeared. So, considerable volume of liquids should be consumed in order to provide frequent fluid replenishment in the urinary tract. The person of anyone in the family suffered nephrolithiasis, or the anatomical defect occurred, represents the higher risk to suffer nephrolithiasis.

**Is professional activity influencing nephrolithiasis risk?**

Another question concerns the age of nephrolithiasis appearance in relation to one's professional activity. We analyse 4 professions (see the questionnaire) and compare the age. (It has been stated that the age distribution in all professional groups is normal distribution). In that situation, applying the ANOVA test will answer whether one's professional activity has any connection with the age of nephrolithiasis appearance in the urinary system.

| PROFESSION | AGE (years) | | | TEST applied | p | H₀ | DECISION |
|---|---|---|---|---|---|---|---|
| | n | $\bar{x}$ | s | | | | |
| MINER | 44 | 48.9 | 8.3 | ANOVA | 0.001 | REJECT | DIFFERENCES SIGNIFICANT |
| COOK | 21 | 46.5 | 10.9 | | | | |
| SPORTSMAN | 12 | 27.1 | 6.4 | BONFERRONI | | 1–3 2–3 4–3 | SIGNIFICANT DIFFERENCES BETWEEN GROUPS |
| OTHER | 143 | 51.2 | 16.1 | | | | |

**Tab. 9.2.** The result table of the ANOVA. The left part of table shows the descriptive statistics. The right part of the table presents the result of statistical tests application: ANOVA and post hoc Bonferroni test distinguishing groups of significant difference between average age in particular group

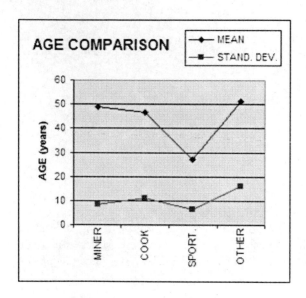

**Fig. 9.2.** The graphic presentation of mean age differentiation in groups and standard deviation in groups of different profession

**Interpretation**

We have found that there is a difference of age (expressed by the arithmetic mean) between the professional groups. Additionally, the *post hoc* (*post factum*) Bonferroni test has pointed those pairs of groups where the difference between them has been essential.

It signifies, that the choice of profession substantially influences the age in which nephrolithiasis can appear. The professions connected with limited drink access, high workplace temperature and high perspiration inducing professions are likely to cause nephrolithiasis appearance in a substantially earlier age than in other professional fields.

**We have already stated that the dietary customs influence the chemical composition of stone in the urinary tract.**

Our diet should be differentiated. One-sided diet enhances the concentration of homogenous chemical compounds, which causes this compound sediment deposition, in the next stage sand formation and eventually large deposits. Providing organism with constant and excessive supply of homogenous nutritive components is likely to bring about an excessive concentration of respective compounds in one's urine and eventually the saturation state excess. Under such circumstances, the deposit appearance is its simple and obvious consequence.

| DIET | CHEMICAL COMPOUND | | | | $\chi^2$ test | | DECISION |
|------|-----------|----------|---------|-------|--------|--------|-----------|
| | PHOSPHATE | URIC AC. | OXALATE | TOTAL | p | $H_0$ | |
| MEAT | 6 | 27 | 31 | 64 | | | |
| DIARY | 34 | 5 | 5 | 44 | 0.0002 | REJECT | DEPENDENCE SIGNIFICANT |
| VEGET. | 21 | 12 | 109 | 142 | | | |
| TOTAL | 61 | 44 | 145 | 250 | | | |

**Tab. 9.3.** The results of $\chi^2$ test applicability estimating the influence of the diet on the chemical compound present in the kidney stone (right part of the table). The contingency table shown in left part of the table

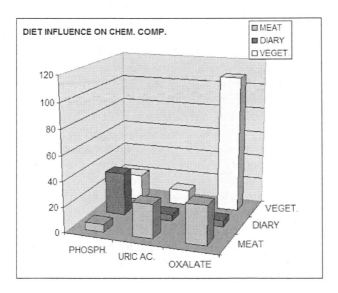

**Fig. 9.3.** The frequencies showing the relation between chemical composition of the deposit and the diet preferred by the patient

**Are the other illnesses influencing nephrolithiasis?**

As these two features: nephrolithiasis character (confined or dispersed) and the circulation disorder presence are qualitative features, the test that can prove their interrelation is $\chi^2$ test.

| NEPHROL. | HEART DISEASE | | | $\chi^2$ test | | DECISION |
|---|---|---|---|---|---|---|
| | PRESENT | ABSENT | TOTAL | p | $H_0$ | |
| CONFINED | 20 | 188 | 208 | | | NO DEPENDENCE |
| DISPERSED | 6 | 24 | 30 | 0.32 | NO REJECT | |
| TOTAL | 26 | 212 | 238 | | | |

**Tab. 9.4.** The summary results of the analysis of the relation between heart disease presence and form of nephrolitiasis (confined or dispersed). Left site presents the contingency table, the right one the $\chi^2$ test results stating absence of any relation between these two variables

**Interpretation**
The heart disease found in the patient with nephrolithiasis have no influence upon the nephrolithiasis character (confined or dispersed).

An analogous analysis was conducted for the other accompanying diseases in relation to confined and dispersed nephrolithiasis. The connection between nephrolithiasis and other illnesses was proved. Osteoporosis, obesity, hypertension, chronic immobilization and primary hyperparathyrosis have a strict connection with the dispersed nephrolithiasis.
The enumerated disease units cause general metabolism disorder in the whole organism, and are the source of faster insoluble sediment deposition. Under such circumstances the primary cause (the accompanying disease) should be treated first, which will result in slowing down the crystallization processes.
It has also been proved that the circulation disorders have no influence upon the nephrolithiasis character (confined or dispersed). It signifies that the circulation disorders and the physiological disorders resulting from them have no metabolic common background with nephrolithiasis.

**Do the disease characteristics depend on the patient's gender?**

That dependence can be stated when analysing the dependence of the stone localization and the examined person's gender. In such circumstances we refer to the $\chi^2$ independence test, as both features are qualitative. We construct the contingency table in which the rows express gender and the columns show localization. The results of such analysis are presented in the table below:

| GENDER | LOCALIZATION | | | | $\chi^2$ test | | DECISION |
|---|---|---|---|---|---|---|---|
| | KIDNEY | URETER | BLADDER | TOTAL | p | $H_0$ | |
| F | 50 | 39 | 5 | 94 | | | DEPENDENCE SIGNIFICANT |
| M | 117 | 31 | 15 | 163 | 0.0002 | REJECT | |
| TOTAL | 167 | 70 | 20 | 257 | | | |

**Tab. 9.5.** The table of results of dependence analysis between the patient's gender and the deposit localization. Such a dependence was proved to exist

## Interpretation

Statistically significant dependence between the patient's gender and the deposit localization was found.

It can be concluded that the differences in the anatomical structure of the urinary tract in men and women are connected with urine retention in the respective parts of the urinary tract.

### Does the presence of certain accompanying diseases influence the stone localization?

Prostate hypertrophy is a frequent disease of urinary tract in men. Let us ask, then, if the disease influences the age in which nephrolithiasis appears?
We analyse two patients' groups: with present or absent prostate hypertrophy and we compare the age of patients in those two groups. In such a situation (after the earlier finding of normal distribution that describes the age distribution of both groups compared) we shall conduct the t-Student test. The results obtained are presented in the table below.

| PROSTATE HYPETROPHY | AGE (years) | | | TEST applied | p | $H_0$ | DECISION |
|---|---|---|---|---|---|---|---|
| | n | $\bar{x}$ | s | | | | |
| ABSENT | 136 | 48.5 | 12.3 | F | 0.06 | No rejection | Dispersion – no differences |
| PRESENT | 26 | 76.00 | 10.1 | t | 0.001 | REJECT | Mean values – difference significant |

**Tab. 9.6.** The summary of the t-Student test application to analyze the significance between mean age values of patients with/without prostate hypertrophy, which appeared to be significant although no difference has been found for age dispersion in these two groups

## Interpretation

We have found out that the age of the patient with prostate hypertrophy is substantially different from the medium age of the patient without prostate hypertrophy.[45]

If one is an elderly man, he should take into account prostate hypertrophy and the following nephrolithiasis connected with urine retention in urinary tract and sedimentation of stones composed of solution-resistant compound salts.

One can be anxious though that the dependence pointed above is connected only with age. In order to make the analysis more precise, we shall ask a question specific to prostate hypertrophy.

### Does prostate hypertrophy influence the stone localization?

For that purpose we reach for the information concerning the localization of the stone, dividing the patients according to the sediment presence in bladder and prostate hypertrophy found. We analyse two qualitative features, so we again refer to the $\chi^2$ independence test. In that case we slightly modify the data base by defining the new variable (the procedure shown in the workbook part), according to which we shall differentiate only the localization within the bladder and other localization (putting together the ureter and the kidney). The analysis will be conducted only for men (the filtration procedure).

The results are given in the table below:

| PROSTATE HYPERTROPHY | LOCALIZATION IN BLADDER | | | $\chi^2$ test | | DECISION |
|---|---|---|---|---|---|---|
| | NO | YES | TOTAL | p | $H_0$ | |
| PRESENT | 12 | 14 | 26 | | | DEPENDENCE SIGNIFICANT |
| ABSENT | 131 | 5 | 136 | 0.0002 | REJECT | |
| TOTAL | 143 | 19 | 162 | | | |

**Tab. 9.7.** The result summary of analyzing the localization in bladder relation to the presence of prostate hypertrophy, which appeared to be significant. Left part of the table presents the contingency table with frequencies and right one presenting the results of $\chi^2$ test applicability

## Interpretation

We have found that prostate hypertrophy really influences the stone localization in the bladder. If the prostate hypertrophy is found in a patient, it can be expected that if a stone appears in the urinary tract, it can be assumed with a high probability that it will be localized the bladder.

---

[45] Another example of applying the one-sided t-Student test. Mind that the complete group numerical strength had been limited to the number of men. This example is also a good one-sided test illustration.

Osteoporosis is another illness also connected with age. It remains in a close connection with calcium salts regulation in bones. It can also be connected with different than regular concentration of calcium salts in urine. Let us ask a question, then:

**What is the age characteristics of the people with osteoporosis found?**

We divide the patients into two groups: with the found osteoporosis and the group free from osteoporosis occurrence. The comparison concerns the medium age of the two groups. We are going to perform the t-Student test (after prior finding the normal distribution as describing the age in both groups).

The results obtained are presented in the table below:

| OSTEOPOROSIS | AGE (years) | | | TEST applied | p | $H_0$ | DECISION |
|---|---|---|---|---|---|---|---|
| | n | $\bar{x}$ | s | | | | |
| PRESENT | 25 | 75.44 | 12.9 | F | 0.24 | No rejection | Dispersion – no differences |
| ABSENT | 205 | 46.85 | 15.8 | t | 0.001 | REJECT | Mean values – difference significant |

**Tab. 9.8.** Test t results stating the difference between the age of people with osteoporosis found in relation to the group of people free from that illness

**Interpretation**
We found that there are elderly people with osteoporosis.[46]
Osteoporosis has proved to concern patients in substantially older age. It has also proved that these patients are women.

Mind that the patients with osteoporosis constitute a relatively numerous group both with respect to the whole sample, and with respect to the number of men, whom another advanced age illness concerned, which is to say prostate hypertrophy.
This observation has a substantial meaning for the complex analysis of our data base of patients with nephrolithiasis. We stated at the very beginning of our analysis, that the age of men represented the distribution comparable to the normal distribution. The distribution of women's age proved to be substantially different from the normal distribution. If the histogram representing the women's age distribution is to be analysed, a high column is observed for high age values class (see histogram Fig. 2.13. and 2.14. in STEP 2 of theory part). The high column represents exactly the women with osteoporosis diagnosed. As that disease concerns a larger number of women than a gender-dependent illness, like it is the case with prostate hypertrophy with men (at least in our

---

[46] Another example of the one-sided t-Student test application.

analysed sample of patients with nephrolithiasis), that group (women with osteoporo-sis) "distorts" the expected normal distribution of women's age.

Most probably, eliminating women with osteoporosis from the sample analysed would cause an approximation of women's age distribution to normal distribution.

The above examples indicate that nephrolithiasis can be avoided if the coexisting ill-nesses are cured.

### Is secluded and dispersed urolithiasis connected with other diagnosed illnesses?

The nephrolithiasis connected with other accompanying illnesses has been reported also for the dependence of dispersed nephrolithiasis on accompanying illnesses ($\chi^2$ – secluded and dispersed nephrolithiasis and the type of accompanying illness). If this discussion is limited to the fact of primary hyperparathyrosis presence or in case of other contingency table for the osteoporosis appearance), it will prove that simultane-ous appearance of nephrolithiasis localized in several places has a strong connection with those illnesses.

As both the primary hyperparathyrosis diagnosing, and the information of secluded or dispersed nephrolithiasis character are qualitative features, the $\chi^2$ independence test is again referred to:

| Nepholithiasis | Primary hiperparathyrosis | | | $\chi^2$ test | | DECISION |
|---|---|---|---|---|---|---|
| | PRESENT | ABSENT | TOTAL | p | H$_0$ | |
| SECLUDED | 5 | 200 | 205 | | | SIGNIFICANT DIFFERENCES |
| DISPERSED | 16 | 35 | 51 | 0.0001 | REJECT | |
| TOTAL | 21 | 235 | 256 | | | |

**Tab. 9.9.** The table presents the results of $\chi^2$ test analysing the dependence between the confined and dispersed nephrolithiasis and other disease, which is the primary hyperparathyrosis. The left side of table shows the contingency table, the right site summarizes the result of the $\chi^2$ test ap-plied for the data shown in left part of the table

### Interpretation

A substantial dependence has been stated between the kind of nephrolithiasis (secluded and dispersed) and the accompanying disease, the primary hyperparathyrosis.

We shall further ask if osteoporosis also has a connection with the nephrolithiasis char-acter (secluded or dispersed) also performing the $\chi^2$ independence test.

| NEPHROLITIASIS | OSTEOPOROSIS | | | $\chi^2$ test | | DECISION |
|---|---|---|---|---|---|---|
| | PRESENT | ABSENT | TOTAL | p | $H_0$ | |
| SECLUDED | 9 | 196 | 205 | | | SIGNIFICANT DIFFERENCES |
| DISPERSED | 16 | 35 | 51 | 0.0001 | REJECT | |
| TOTAL | 25 | 231 | 256 | | | |

**Tab. 9.10.** The table presenting the results of $\chi^2$ test stating the dependence between the nephrolithiasis form (secluded and dispersed) and the fact of osteoporosis appearance

## Interpretation

The osteoporosis presence has a substantial influence upon the nephrolithiasis character (secluded and dispersed).

Summing up we can state that the diseases that cause changing the general metabolic system processes cause generation of crystalline deposits regardless their localization. At an enhanced mobilizing of calcium from bones, its concentration grows in the organic fluids causing calcium salts crystallising in urine tracts.
Anatomical changes in a specific urine tract part cause the appearance of a crystalline deposit in the anatomically deformed area. However, a general organic distortion in calcium salts distribution causes the appearance of deposits in dispersed localization.

It has already been told that the deposit localization in the case of defined anatomical disorder within the urinary system influences the stone localization and differentiates it.

The question:

**Does the specified anatomical disorder influence the stone localization?**

Will be answered by performing the $\chi^2$ independence test (both qualitative features):

| LOCALIZATION | Anatomical defects | | | | $\chi^2$ test | | DECISION |
|---|---|---|---|---|---|---|---|
| | PO | PD | SK | TOTAL | p | $H_0$ | |
| KIDNEY | 61 | 26 | 4 | 91 | | | TEST NOT APPLIED |
| URETER | 27 | 19 | 1 | 47 | | | |
| BLADDER | 2 | 3 | 1 | 6 | | | |
| TOTAL | 90 | 48 | 6 | 144 | | | |

**Tab. 9.11.a.** The $\chi^2$ test results depicting the presence of dependence between the stone localization and the kind of anatomical disorder. The $\chi^2$ test can not be applied due to low frequencies in one column and one row

| LOCALIZATION | Anatomical defects | | | $\chi^2$ test | | DECISION |
|---|---|---|---|---|---|---|
| | PO | PD | TOTAL | p | H$_0$ | |
| KIDNEY | 61 | 26 | 87 | | NO REJECT | NO DEPENDENCE |
| URETER | 27 | 19 | 46 | 18.55 | | |
| TOTAL | 88 | 45 | 133 | | | |

**Tab. 9.11.b.** The $\chi^2$ test results depicting the presence of dependence between the stone localization and the kind of anatomical disorder after the removal of cases of the frequencies lower than 5. The calculation was performed with these patients excluded, although if there is any reason to incorporate them to another class, it can be done also
PO – Pyelocalyceal obstruction, PD – Pyelocalyceal duplication, SK – Spongeous kidney

## Interpretation
There is a statistically significant dependence between the stone localization and the anatomical defect type.

The above statement signifies that a specific anatomical defect has a specific influence upon the distortion in urine flow and its retention in the strictly specified places of the urine tract.
Coming back to the previous analysis, the general organic distortion in calcium salts distribution does not influence local distortion in the flow and retention of urine in the specific localization.
However, an anatomical change influences the deposit localization as it locally distorts urine circulation and makes a retention site that enables crystallization.

Coming back to the problems of possible anatomical defect inheritance, one could ask another question:

**Does the family interview indicating nephrolithiasis in the family members have a connection with the specific anatomical defect?**

As both the analysed features are qualitative, we shall perform the $\chi^2$ independence test:

| FAMILY INTERVIEW | Anatomical defects | | | | $\chi^2$ test | | DECISION |
|---|---|---|---|---|---|---|---|
| | PO | PD | SK | TOTAL | p | H$_0$ | |
| PRESENT | 85 | 47 | 5 | 137 | | | |
| ABSENT | 7 | 5 | 1 | 13 | | | NOT APPLIED |
| TOTAL | 92 | 52 | 6 | 150 | | | |

**Tab. 9.12.a.** Finding the dependence between the anatomical defect type and the fact of nephrolithiasis appearance in the family. The condition for the $\chi^2$ test applicability not satisfied due to low frequencies in the SK column

| FAMILY INTERVIEW | Anatomical defects | | | $\chi^2$ test | | DECISION |
|---|---|---|---|---|---|---|
| | PO | PD | TOTAL | p | $H_0$ | |
| PRESENT | 85 | 47 | 132 | | | NO DEPENDENCE |
| ABSENT | 7 | 5 | 12 | 0.67 | NO REJECT | |
| TOTAL | 92 | 52 | 144 | | | |

**Tab. 9.12.b.** Finding the dependence between the anatomical defect type and the fact of nephrolithiasis appearance in the family. The removal of the column containing the low frequencies made possible the $\chi^2$ test applicable

**Interpretation**
We have stated that there is no dependence between the anatomical defect type and the family interview itself.

Although we have stated no dependence between the family interview (the persons with a diagnosed anatomical defect present in the patient's family) and the type of the anatomical defect, in our interpretation it indicates the fact, that regardless of the defect, it is transferred to the young generation.
If we know of anybody in our family (parents, grandparents, siblings), that they suffered from nephrolithiasis for the anatomical defects (regardless of the defect type) we can expect that the disease will concern us, too.

Continuing with the anatomical analysis, we shall ask:

**Does nephrolithiasis appear in a comparable age regardless the anatomical defects?**

We refer to the ANOVA test again. We are going to analyse three groups (different anatomical defects) from the point of view if the anatomical defect type. Mean patient's age is compared in those groups, thus a measurable feature. The arrangement of analysed features justifies the ANOVA test conducting, provided the normal distribution is represented in all the analysed groups.

| ANATOMIC DEFECT | AGE (years) | | | TEST applied | p | $H_0$ | DECISION |
|---|---|---|---|---|---|---|---|
| | n | $\bar{x}$ | s | | | | |
| PO | 48 | 34.5 | 8.3 | ANOVA | 0.12 | NO REJECT | NO DIFFERENCES |
| PD | 80 | 37.4 | 10.9 | | | | |
| SK | 6 | 35.0 | 6.4 | BONFERRONI | | NOT PER-FORMED | |

**Tab. 9.13.** The results of applying the ANOVA test to find the absence of differences between the age in which renal nephrolithiasis appears in the groups of people with a specific urinary system anatomical defect

## Interpretation
No differences were found between the mean values of age in the compared groups (obtained for the type of anatomical defect).

It signifies that all the anatomical defects "accelerate" the nephrolithiasis appearance in a comparable degree.

If we ask another question:

**Does nephrolithiasis really appear earlier in the people with the diagnosed anatomical defect?**

We shall conduct the t-Student test for this purpose

| ANATOMIC DEFECT | AGE (years) | | | TEST applied | p | $H_0$ | DECISION |
|---|---|---|---|---|---|---|---|
| | n | $\bar{x}$ | s | | | | |
| ABSENT | 105 | 52.8 | 11.6 | F | 0.001 | REJECT | Dispersion – differences SIGNIFICANT |
| PRESENT | 151 | 38.3 | 24.3 | t | 0.001 | REJECT | Mean values – difference SIGNIFICANT |

**Tab. 9.14.** The results of conducted test t comparing the mean age of persons with and without the diagnosed congenital patient's defect

## Interpretation
It has been stated that nephrolithiasis really appears earlier in the persons with the diagnosed anatomical defect.

Continuing the issue problem of accompanying diseases influence upon the nephrolithiasis appearance, we shall ask a question:

**Does the appearance of nephrolithiasis take place in a substantially earlier age in the case of diagnosed primary hyperparathyrosis?**

This question will be answered by the t-Student test for two groups (diagnosed primary hyperparathyrosis YES, NO – two groups), and we shall analyze the mean age values (a measurable feature):

| HYPER PARATHYROSIS | AGE (years) | | | TEST applied | p | $H_0$ | DECISION |
|---|---|---|---|---|---|---|---|
| | n | $\bar{x}$ | s | | | | |
| ABSENT | 242 | 48.34 | 17.8 | F | 0.01 | REJECT | Dispersion – differences SIGNIFICANT |
| PRESENT | 7 | 36.57 | 10.5 | t | 0.01 | REJECT | Mean values – difference SIGNIFICANT |

**Tab. 9.15.** The significance of age difference of the appearance of nephrolithiasis among the persons, in whom primary hyperparathyrosis was or was not found

**Interpretation**
The diagnosed primary hyperparathyrosis causes the nephrolithiasis appearance in the substantially earlier age.

Generalizing all the results concerning the coexisting illnesses it can be stated, that the enumerated anatomical defects and general system metabolism distortions concerning the distribution of calcium salts belong to the factors accelerating nephrolithiasis appearance.

The obtained results, constituting the examples of using tests depending on the form of information recording and concerning relation analysis between the increased calcium salts concentration and the fact of osteoporosis appearance are the following:

The test t-Student comparing the medium concentrations of calcium salts in patients' urine in two groups of people with diagnosed osteoporosis and without it produced the following results:

| OSTEOPOROSIS | CONCENTRATION OF $Ca^{2+}$ (mmol/l) | | | TEST applied | p | $H_0$ | DECISION |
|---|---|---|---|---|---|---|---|
| | n | $\bar{x}$ | s | | | | |
| ABSENT | 249 | 3.4 | 0.7 | F | 0.01 | REJECT | Dispersion – differences SIGNIFICANT |
| PRESENT | 7 | 6.7 | 1.2 | t | 0.01 | REJECT | Mean values – difference SIGNIFICANT |

**Tab. 9.16.** The results of testing the difference significance of calcium salts between the group of people with diagnosed osteoporosis and the people with whom the disease was not found

**Interpretation**

A significant difference was found in the concentration of calcium salts in the persons with and without osteoporosis.

The same question can be analysed on the basis of the newly introduced variable called WG expressing the affiliation to the group with excessive calcium salts level in urine considered normal. This time we are analysing two qualitative features we refer to the chi-square independence test then. The results obtained are the following:

| $Ca^{2+}$ CONCENTRATION ABOVE THE STANDARD ONE $> 5$ mmol/l | OSTEOPOROSIS | | | $\chi^2$ test | | DECISION |
|---|---|---|---|---|---|---|
| | PRESENT | ABSENT | TOTAL | p | $H_0$ | |
| YES | 6 | 18 | 24 | | | SIGNIFICANT DIFFERENCES |
| NO | 5 | 227 | 232 | 0.001 | REJECT | |
| TOTAL | 11 | 245 | 256 | | | |

**Tab. 9.17.** The results of $\chi^2$ test stating the dependence between the fact of osteoporosis diagnosis fact and the fact of exceeding calcium salts concentration considered normal

**Interpretation**

We rejected the $H_0$ of $\chi^2$ test which signifies that there is a statistically significant connection between the fact of enhanced calcium salts concentration in urine and the osteoporosis presence. It signifies that ubnormal calcium salts distribution (bone degradation processes) influences the excess of calcium salts concentration in urine considered normal.

Summing up the last two analyses it should be admitted that information interesting to us can be obtained on the basis of various data. The selection is dictated by the character and type of data that we have at our disposal in the given situation.

## CORRELATION – REGRESSION ANALYSIS

As was stated earlier, pH value is a very simple and very cheep measurement and not invasive analysis. This is why we would like to explore as much as possible the information carried by the pH value. The question which may be asked is whether its value correlates with any another measurements. The correlation between pH and $Ca^{2+}$ as well as $Mg^{2+}$ concentrations was found to be proportional and significant. It means that the higher ions concentration the higher pH value. Meanwhile the correlation between pH and the number of erythrocyte appears not to be significant. The appropriate coefficients for regression functions appeared to be significant for $Ca^{2+}$ versus pH and $Mg^{2+}$ versus pH. Meanwhile the regression parameters for pH and number of erythrocytes appeared to be not statistically significant. It means, that the pressure of erythrocytes has nothing in common with acidity of urine.

## THE SUMMARY OF COMPREHENSIVE ANALYSIS

Our knowledge upon the solubility of inorganic salts teaches us (which we actually presented in the chapter *Correlation and Regression*), that the only way of preventing from exceeding the threshold salt concentration value in the solution is diluting it. The basic means of prevention, then, consists in enhancing the quantity of drinks consumed in 24 hours.

We stated also, that there were independent factors:

1.  Whose presence we are able to influence: profession, diet,
2.  And those, that we are unable to control:

     A – general organic – the calcium salts distribution distortion;

     B – local – anatomical defects.


A factor that we are able to influence is the suitable occupation choice. A profession that includes a limited access to drinks is a factor that creates favourable conditions to nephrolithiasis in our organism. The choice of a profession connected with intensive perspiration is also risky for people with nephrolithiasis predisposition.

Another factor that we can influence is the kind of diet. Each one-sided diet may cause the increase in specified mineral salts concentration. We stated that relation when we proved that a different stone composition corresponds to a different chemical composition of stone. If our diet is balanced, no salt will exceed the critical concentration and no deposit of a given chemical composition will appear.

The predisposition appears in the family interview, that indicates the nephrolithiasis occurrence in the family or the presence of possible anatomical defects within the urinary system.

We also pointed out that metabolism disturbing could cause appearance of crystalline deposits in many locations of the urinary tract.

The accompanying diseases connected with age (osteoporosis, prostate hypertrophy) substantially create favourable conditions for stone formation in urinary tract.


Genetic conditioning can be the least influenced among the enumerated factors. Although, if they had already been found, one should carefully consider the appropriate occupation choice. The profession that may in any way influence our excessive perspiration (high temperatures) limiting the access to drinks (astronauts, and in the future spaceship passengers) should not be recommended to people with urinary tract anatomical defects.

If we were diagnosed any illnesses like: osteoporosis, primary hyperparathyrosis, prostate hypertrophy (and the other enumerated above), which (as it was indicated) influence the urinary tract stone appearance, first of all the causal disease should be treated.

The easiest way, as it seems, is to protect oneself from nephrolithiasis keeping an appropriate diet. Either $Ca^{2+}$ rich (dairy), or meat based diet (causing excessive uric acid concentration) seem to influence the increase in concentration of mineral salts that cause specific ailments if they crystallize in the urinary system.

All those factors are joined with one superior message, to consume an appropriate volume of liquids. An adequate volume of liquids in the daily diet will directly influence the components of urine that bear a threat that their crystalline form will appear.

The presented complex analysis was supposed to envisage that the subsequently asked detailed questions concerning particular phenomena and in complex arrangement in relation to an adequate statistical test help to obtain an answer of a more general character. A set of narrowly specified particular issues enables, applying general knowledge, draw one or more conclusions (in proportion to the number of particular information – in our example) of general nature. If another patient sees us, whom we ask basic questions about his or her working conditions and associate them with the age (and gender), it will be possible to provide applying adequate medical means.

To sum it up, one can say that there are factors that we can influence (choosing the profession, kind of diet, lifestyle) and those that result from the urinary system anatomical structure or inappropriate metabolism (frequently resulting from the pathological processes with no direct correspondence to the urinary system).
So, if an non-optimal anatomical structure was found in us (family interview), we should not make things worse by choosing a profession unfavourable for us in that arrangement (we should not accept a limited access to liquids and considerable physical effort).
If we suffer from other illnesses, that eventually influence inappropriate metabolism and mineral distribution (primary hyperparathyrosis, osteoporosis), those illnesses should be cured which causes higher concentration of salts that easily form deposit (crystallize) in urine.

Giving further examples of detailed questions and presenting appropriate statistical tests that can help in problem solution if used properly.
Choosing the right test, one should take into account the characteristics of analysed (compared) features. It is also important to specify the compared groups in a clear and definite way. The criterion of dividing into appropriate groups should be precisely defined and attention focused on the point where, in which question (which feature) the criterion to sub-group division is contained.
It has also been shown how to transform the data in order to obtain the desired final result changing the given feature's status. It has been shown how to eliminate (at full realizing the reasons for this elimination) those study results (those persons) who would, in the given, specific situation, disintegrate the final results.
We can obtain precious information upon the conducted diagnostics, therapy or prevention by asking a question in the right way, referring to the right data, and using an appropriate statistical test.
Statistical methods in medicine are helpful accessory tools for data analysis, describing samples that represent adequate groups of people suffering from specific ailments.

# Exercises

1. Try to ask a series of questions about:

   A – the objective causes of death (The patient's age – does it influence the survival, in other words, is the age of the dead really higher than the age of survivors? What test specifies it?);

   B – the accident circumstances induced causes of death – in relation to the casualty's role (a cyclist, a pedestrian, etc.) and in relation to the distance from the closest emergency ambulance service or hospital;

   C – was the first operation term connected with the patient's death (Was an average time of waiting for the operation substantially longer with the deceased than with the survivors?);

   D – health condition evaluation upon leaving the hospital – is impairment percentage (%) related to age? or to treatment duration? or to multiple injuries?

2. Do you think that other questions should have been asked in the questionnaire? If so, suggest the way of information record extension and its storage.

3. Try to suggest a set of questions, appropriate tests and data to be used if you want to make an analysis from the point of view of:

   A – a therapeutic procedures applied for patients in emergency medicine and multiple trauma;

   B – senior registrar of the ward – equipment supply (e.g. the number of patients that need rehabilitation equipment) and the adequate personnel number (extra help needed) depending on the day of the week – accidents number different on different days;

   C – insurance provider – the casualties' age, impairment frequency and character, etc.;

   D – sociological and demographic analysis (social status of the casualties, accidents in and outside the workplace).

# STEP 9 – exercise

# COMPREHENSIVE ANALYSIS

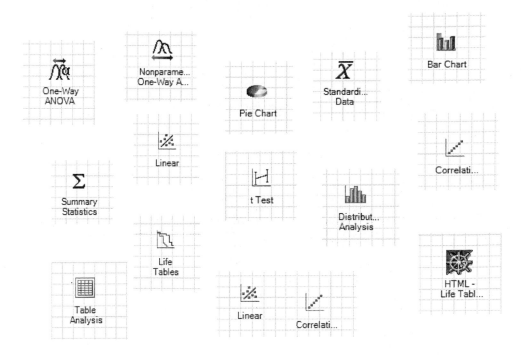

A set of questions about a specific medical problem is always rich. You may also ask questions about a selected group of subjects in our database. You may choose only those who died and in the next step those who survived (it is not our case but the problem is frequently analyzed in medical science). Going back to our database, you may for instance select those who are vegetarian to find out some, if any, differences with respect to those who prefer other types of diet.

You may analyze patients with diabetes as a concomitant disease and compare them with patients having urolithiasis.
We use various tests in a comprehensive analysis. The choice depends on the nature of data. There are tests which are used many times; other tests may not be used at all.

**Remember, that statistical analysis is a tool for solving a medical problem. The problem itself (and an appropriate set of data) decides about the set of statistical tests to be used.**

Below you will find a representation of the process of analysis to use Student's t-test where you have to define the type of distribution of a specific feature in the two groups being compared.
Data analysis – Student's t-test

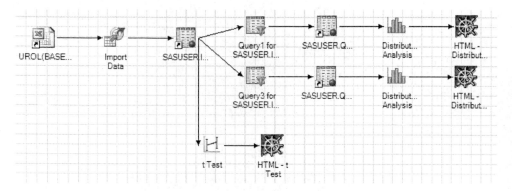

**Fig. 9.1.** Representation of the process of analysis to use Student's t-test. Please note that for each of the groups being compared the type of distribution has to be defined. Student's t-test can only be performed if all the variables are proved to fit the normal distribution

The scheme above shows a series of consecutive steps to perform appropriately Student's t-test.

Double filtering ("Query") is done to identify two groups to perform independent analyses of distribution ("Distribut... Analysis"). The results of the distribution analysis are saved as sets under the icons "HTML Distribut...".
If the feature in both groups fits the normal distribution, we go back to the complete database and perform Student's t-test. The results of this analysis are available upon activation of the icon "HTML t-Test".

ANOVA TEST

The ANOVA test also requires that the normality assumptions are met. For this reason distribution analysis should be repeated for each group being compared at a specific step of our analysis.
The correctly performed procedure for the ANOVA test is shown below when comparing three groups.

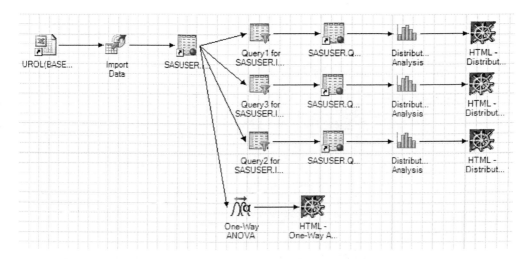

**Fig. 9.2.** Complete ANOVA test to compare three groups taking into account distribution analysis in each group

The normality assumptions were tested three times. The result sets (represented by the icon "HTML Distribut...") provide the information that the feature (for instance urinary pH) analyzed in each group defined by one factor (for instance stone location) fits the normal distribution. Only then we go back to the primary database (complete) and perform the ANOVA test to compare the means of the quantifiable features in three groups.

Summing up the information regarding parametric tests (see the scheme STEP 5 theory part Fig. 5.2), the normality assumptions must be met and they should be tested before any parametric analyses are carried out.

CONTINGENCY TABLE ANALYSIS

Below you will find a typical procedure to carry out a $\chi^2$ test. As you may see, there are no conditions that should be met before the analysis.

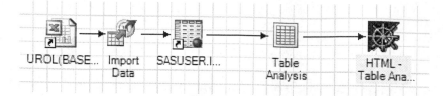

**Fig. 9.3.** Representation of the analysis of contingency table (dependence between qualitative features)

Only when it is justified to eliminate temporarily some records (for instance too small sample size), the testing is preceded by the filtering.

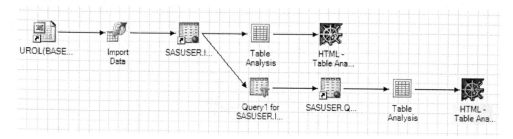

**Fig. 9.4.** If the numbers of records in the contingency table are too small, such groups should be eliminated as the result of the test would be distorted

The scheme above shows the consecutive steps to perform the analysis of dependence between the qualitative features when it was necessary to filter the data.

There are some operations on the data that require our attention:

## DECLARATION OF A NEW FEATURE (QUALITATIVE) DEFINED ON THE BASIS OF ANOTHER (QUANTITATIVE) FEATURE

We mentioned before that it is possible to transform quantitative measurements into qualitative values. It is obvious that some information is lost in this process as we get only a qualitative classification of the feature measured before. Below you will find an example of such analysis.

Let's take urinary calcium content. We ask a question whether the content of urinary calcium salts in patents with osteoporosis is significantly higher than in patients without osteoporosis.

In this situation we perform Student's t-test to compare the mean content of calcium salts in patients with and without osteoporosis. Below you will find two table columns with the data to perform the analysis.[47]

| ● CaC | ♣ OSTEOP# |
|---|---|
| 7.18 | Y |
| 4.31 | N |
| 3.28 | N |
| 0.56 | N |
| 6.23 | Y |
| 5.81 | Y |
| 6.37 | Y |
| 0.88 | N |
| 1.44 | N |
| 2.09 | N |
| 2.87 | N |
| 4.32 | N |
| 3.31 | N |

**Fig. 9.5.** Data on calcium salt content in the urine and presence or absence of osteoporosis in females

Our data analysis spreadsheet has two columns: one with urinary calcium content (mmol/l) and another stating whether osteoporosis is present or absent.

Another analysis regarding the relationship between urinary calcium content and osteoporosis may be performed after categorization of patients by the magnitude of calcium content (the variable CaC). In other words, the information on calcium content may become qualitative. Calcium content below 5 mmol/l is normal and provides the information that the metabolic processes are normal. Calcium content > 5 mmol/l indicates that the metabolism of calcium is disordered. The patients may be then subdivided into those below and above the cutoff value. We introduce a new feature CA. As a result we get a new feature in a new column. This operation prepares you to perform a $\chi^2$ test analysis for two qualitative features (presence of osteoporosis and calcium content above the normal level in urine). The $\chi^2$ test will answer a question whether there is a relationship between osteoporosis and excess calcium content.

Below you will find the steps to construct a new feature based on another (quantitative) one.

---

[47] Based on the former analysis on the occurrence of osteoporosis in women and men, our analysis may be limited only to females.

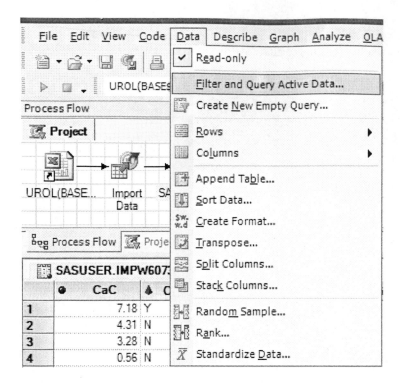

**Fig. 9.6.** Begin with the filtering procedure to introduce a new (qualitative) feature based on the quantitative value

By choosing the "Filter and Query Active Data" you obtain a dialog box in which you have to define further options.

| | Filter Data | **Select and Sort** | Tables | Group Filters | Advanced | Parameters | |
|---|---|---|---|---|---|---|---|
| Σ | | | Item | | ↑↓ | Sort Priority | ∧ |
| ✓ | | | CaC | | | | |
| ✓ | | | OSTEOP# | | | | |
| ✓ | | | GENDER | | | | |

New...

Properties...

**Fig. 9.7.** Dialog box to declare a new variable where we enter codes to define the elevated and normal calcium content in the urine

Choose the "New" button to get a new column.

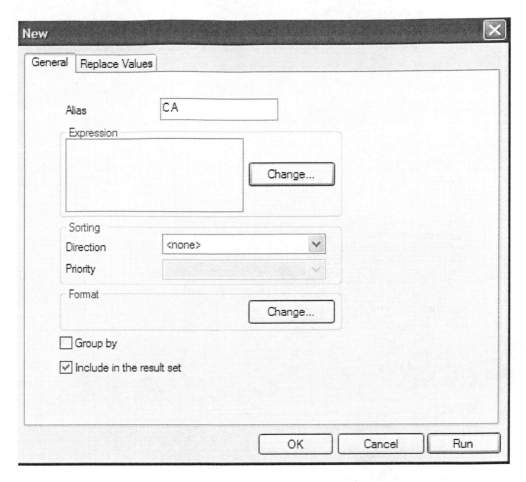

**Fig. 9.8.** Definition of a new variable (coded) CA to express the elevated or normal calcium content in the urine

After declaring the new feature (CA), you specify the conditions for coding calcium content in the qualitative form in the „Expression Builder" dialog box.

By clicling on the „Change" button you obtain a new dialog box:

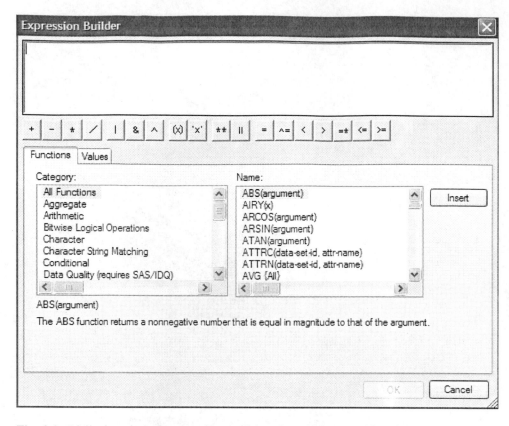

**Fig. 9.9.** Dialog box (upper) to specify conditions by which a specific calcium content is assumed to be elevated or normal

Here you have categories (or operations) that can be used on a given database. In this case we choose "Conditional".

There may be various expressions to define a category. We choose a simple condition „CASE {else}".

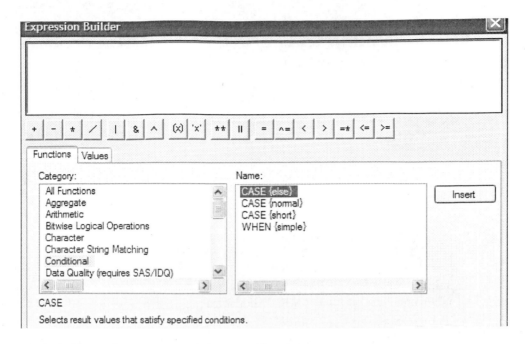

Fig. 9.10. Choose the name to categorize a specific calcium measurement

By choosing this option you go to the upper dialog box where you precisely define the condition.

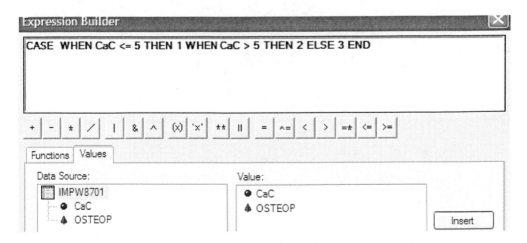

Fig. 9.11. Expression built to specify the condition (using Name and operation symbols)

The expression between < and > should be filled appropriately.

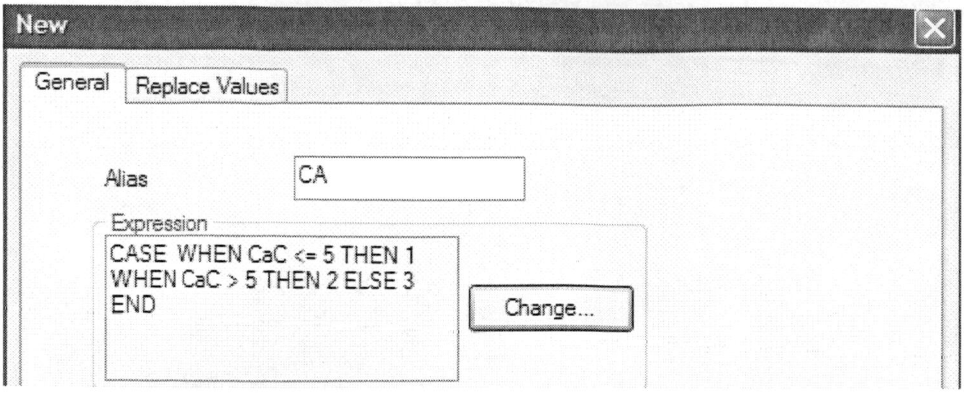

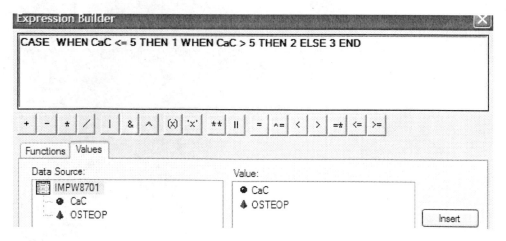

**Fig. 9.12.** Refer to the data in your database

In our example the expression should be filled as follows: If CaC is lower than or equal to 5, the new variable is assumed to be 1. If CaC is higher than 5, the new variable is assumed to be 2, otherwise (for instance if data are absent) the new variable is assumed to be 3. The new feature was declared in the second dialog box of our analysis and for this reason you do not need to state which feature should be coded as defined above. Remember that numbers 1 and 2 (and 3) for the new variable CA do not measure anything. They are used here as codes to categorize subjects with normal (1), elevated (2) calcium content. The code 3 refers to the remaining subjects.

**Fig 9.13.** Correct expression to specify the condition for classification based on quantitative measurement (calcium content in the urine)

The operations above produced a new column named as declared (CA) and coded as defined in our expression.

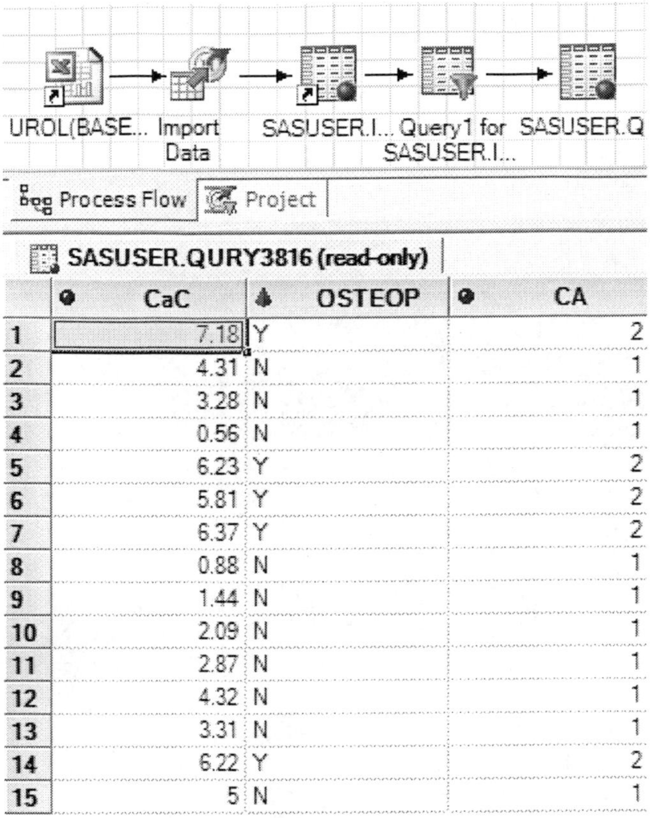

| | CaC | OSTEOP | CA |
|----|------|--------|----|
| 1 | 7.18 | Y | 2 |
| 2 | 4.31 | N | 1 |
| 3 | 3.28 | N | 1 |
| 4 | 0.56 | N | 1 |
| 5 | 6.23 | Y | 2 |
| 6 | 5.81 | Y | 2 |
| 7 | 6.37 | Y | 2 |
| 8 | 0.88 | N | 1 |
| 9 | 1.44 | N | 1 |
| 10 | 2.09 | N | 1 |
| 11 | 2.87 | N | 1 |
| 12 | 4.32 | N | 1 |
| 13 | 3.31 | N | 1 |
| 14 | 6.22 | Y | 2 |
| 15 | 5 | N | 1 |

**Fig. 9.14.** Dialog box with the new qualitative variable

Now you can perform a $\chi^2$ test for two coded features (presence or absence of osteoporosis and classification of subjects by elevated calcium content in the urine). You may ask a question whether elevated calcium content is associated with osteoporosis. You choose the feature "OSTEOPOROSIS" and "CA" to include in the contingency table.

The results of the present analysis in both forms (i.e. Student's t-test to compare the mean calcium content in subjects with and without osteoporosis and $\chi^2$ test to analyze the relationship between osteoporosis and calcium content higher than the normal value) are presented in the main book in STEP 9.

If you need help, it is available by clicking the option "Help" or the icon with a question mark.

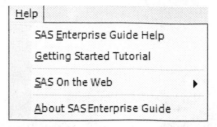

**Fig. 9.15.** Dialog box „Help" and hints available on the toolbar. You may choose a question or search using a key word

We wish you success when using the SAS package.
We hope that failures will be as rare as possible.

We believe that the icon representing the result set will appear each time you expect it to be there.

This is the icon appearing after each successful action.

# STEP 10

# Survival analysis – Is it possible to make prognosis?

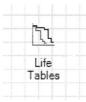

Life
Tables

> **When can we expect the crystalline deposit re-appearance after its removal?**

Survival analysis is one of the methods that have more and more frequently appeared in medical data analyses recently. That analysis introduces a certain novelty element, which consists in a tendency to predict the future, the future course of actions, not necessarily (in spite of the name) connected with the fact of certain survival period itself.

Such analysis deserves defining two medical actions, the first of which is called the initial action (the starting point) and the second one is called the final action (the final point). The starting medical action can be the ailment appearance, including certain phenomena critical for the patient's health and life, e.g. a heart attack, a cerebral haemorrhage or cancer diagnosis. The final action can be not only death, but also a metastasis appearance, another heart attack or any other cardiac trouble. It is important that both the opening (starting), and the final action are explicitly defined for the whole patients group. In order to enable the following analysis performance, the time limits information is also needed. In order to continue the subject started in this handbook, we can ask a question: what is the prognosis in the nephrolithiasis case? The surgical stone removal from the patient's kidney will be assumed as the starting action, while the end point is the stone reappearance expressed with another necessity to operate (at the same localization).[48]

The starting and end points for patients treated with lithotripsy are the first and repeated treatment.

The required precise information concerning the dates of the first and the second deposit removal from the same kidney is rather difficult to obtain because of a long time elapsed between the two operations of stone removal from the same place. If we agree that an adequately long-time patients' observation is possible, two possibilities should be assumed:

1. We know both dates – date of the first operation and the date of reappearance, and

2. We know the date of the first operation (starting event), we observe the patient for some time, and then we practically lose contact as the patient fails to report for routine examination.

3. The patient is under observation and the reappearance did not happen.

The first case is specified as finished observation – graphically signed as a filled circle in the diagram below (a specific state, i.e. the final action has been accomplished).

The second case is specified as a censored observation (the empty circle in the diagram below) (see also the questionnaire given in STEP 1).

The third case is classified as finished observation with no reappearance.

---

[48] The example was chosen only for the calculation method description and to continue the medical problem. The analysis is meaningful for the survival evaluation after heart transplantation, cerebral hemorrhage and other medical events critical for patient's life.

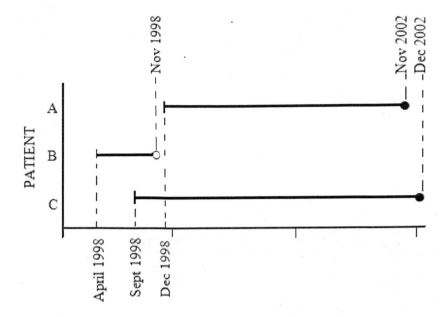

**Fig. 10.1.** The observation period of three sample patients (A, B, C), with whom the operation of stone removal from urinary tract had been performed and another one was necessary because of the stone reappearance. (Time periods given are abbreviated for the higher picture legibility). The empty circle signifies a break of contact with patient (a censored observation) while the filled one signifies the stone resumption

Patient observation time (real time) is presented as in Fig. 10.1.
Many patients' compilation in relative time scale is shown in Fig. 10.2.

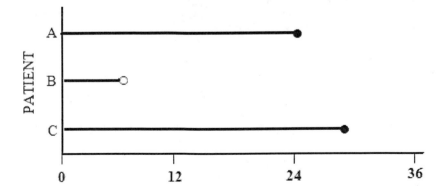

**Fig. 10.2.** Relative survival times, free from a repeated operation necessity. Patient B not observed after ca 6 months since the first operation

Fig. 10.3. is showing the same data in the probability scale of meeting the patient who had no necessity to have the new operation performed (no stone resumption). As it can be seen, in the beginning, just after the operation, no patient expressed a new operation necessity. However, with time elapsed the line in lowers towards the probability scale which signifies that several patients had already needed the new operation of stone removal. We do not know, however, if the line situation was lowered in connection with another operation, or if the patients broke contact with us. That differentiation is visualised as a circle that shows a drop in probability values, resulting mainly from the lack of contact with patients.

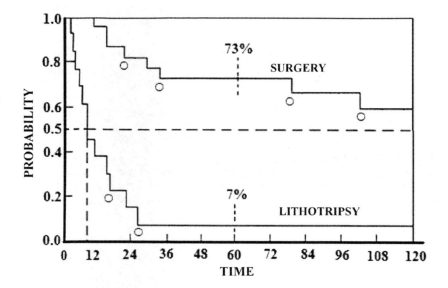

**Fig. 10.3.** Survival times free from the new operation necessity (surgical operation and lithotripsy).The relative numbers of patients (percentage – %) who did not need a repeated surgery for 5 years were marked in the illustration. The time free from operation necessity that half of each of the two analysed patients' groups survives was also marked

**Kaplan-Meier curve** (as the diagram shown in Fig.10.3. is called) can be interpreted in two ways. Two parameters can be read from it (Fig. 10.3.):

1. Survival probability of half the 5-year period (at 5 years' survival defined as recovery),

2. Specifying the time survived by half the observed group without final recovery as 0.5 probability value.

Result presentation with Kaplan-Meier curve enables the disease progression prognosis. These are, of course, only estimates.

The comparative analysis proves invaluable. We analysed the surgical stone removal from urinary tract. Apart from this method of deposit removal, sound wave deposit crushing has been used lately, hoping that the broken crystal would be washed down with urine.

Compared patient observations according to those two methods indicate higher surgical treatment efficiency.

## Exercises

1. Data provided on the attached CD contain no information (such as dates) needed for conducting the survival analysis, although they can be created individually, by transforming information in the position that specifies the date of death. In this case there are no censored actions (as the patients died in our ward). In this situation one more column has to be added, in which e.g. only digits 1 will appear, signifying the final event (death).[49]
   It becomes possible to perform the survival analysis for the data concerning traffic accidents casualties.
2. Please find two parameters on Kaplan-Meier curve diagram: the percent of people who survive the time of half the maximum time period registered in the data, and the time survived half the analysed patients.
3. Suggest performing an analogous analysis separately for patients with multiple and single injuries.
4. Perform a comparative analysis for the groups enumerated in paragraph 3.
5. Suggest another division into the groups of patients in order to perform a comparative analysis.

---

[49] The procedure of adding a new variable to the data base in SAS was shown in the STEP 9.

# STEP 10 – exercise

# Survival analysis

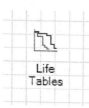

Life
Tables

By clicking on **Analyze** drop-down menu you select **Survival Analysis** and then **Life Tables** options.

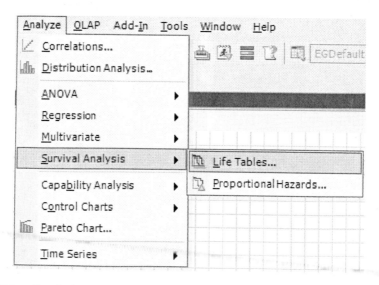

**Fig. 10.1.** Select Survival Analysis from the menu

As usual, you are asked to define the role of a variable.

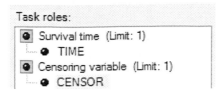

**Fig. 10.2.** Define the variables

In the same dialog box you are asked to code truncated and complete data. If you use symbols other than 0 and 1 to record data, you may enter them in the dialog box below. A tick mark denotes truncated data.

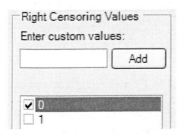

**Fig. 10.3.** Specify the censoring variable. The truncated variable is coded 0

In the next dialog box you select the type of analysis (in this example Kaplan-Meier survival curves) and define the confidence level for survivor function.

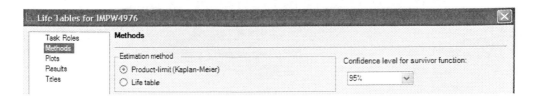

**Fig. 10.4.** Select the Kaplan-Meier survival curves

In another dialog box you select the type of graphic presentation.

**Life Tables for IMPW4976**

Task Roles
Methods
Plots
Results
Titles

**Plots**

☑ Show survival function plot

☑ Include pointwise confidence intervals

☑ Show censored values

**Fig. 10.5.** Specify the type of graphic presentation of the final results

In this example the survival function plot will include confidence intervals and will show censored values.

Plots are shown below. The first plot shows the survival curve, in our case – the time to relapse curve i.e. recurrence of stones requiring intervention (to remove the deposit), with the survival time 0 denoting a first procedure and final time referring to repeat intervention due to recurrence of the primary disease.

The plot includes truncated data (blue balls). The option "Show censored values" (see above) has also been selected.

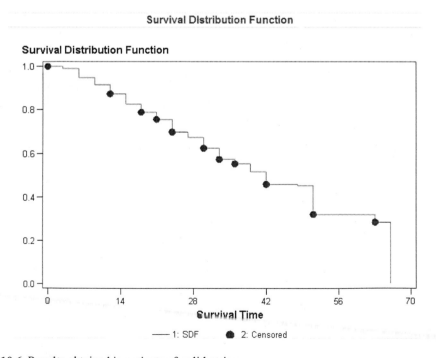

**Fig. 10.6.** Results obtained in patients after lithotripsy

Each patient wants to know the complaint-free time after intervention. The table below contains these parameters. Coming back to quartiles defined in the descriptive statistics, the interpretation is as follows: the first quartile – 75% of the time (17.5 months) without complaints in 66% of patients; 42% of patients survive without complaints 35 months; 24% of patients are complaint free for 52.5 months. The confidence intervals show the limits of error for each estimate.

| Quartile Estimates | | | |
|---|---|---|---|
| | | 95% Confidence Interval | |
| Percent | Point Estimate | [Lower | Upper) |
| 75 | 66.0000 | 63.0000 | 66.0000 |
| 50 | 42.0000 | 36.0000 | 51.0000 |
| 25 | 24.0000 | 18.0000 | 27.0000 |

**Fig. 10.7.** Quartiles (with confidence intervals) for patients after lithotripsy

It is also interesting to know the efficacy of interventions: surgical removal of stones and lithotripsy.
Below is a plot for patients after lithotripsy.

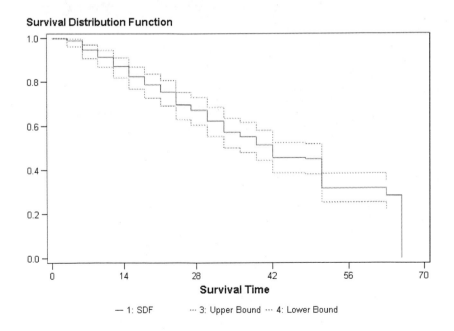

**Fig. 10.8.** Relapse-free survival curve including confidence intervals for patients after lithotripsy

Quartile estimates for complaint-free patients are given below.

| Quartile Estimates | | | |
|---|---|---|---|
| | | 95% Confidence Interval | |
| Percent | Point Estimate | [Lower | Upper) |
| 75 | 66.0000 | 63.0000 | 66.0000 |
| 50 | 42.0000 | 36.0000 | 51.0000 |
| 25 | 24.0000 | 18.0000 | 27.0000 |

**Fig. 10.9.** Quartile estimates and confidence intervals for patients after surgical removal of stones

Below is the survival curve for complaint-free patients after surgical removal of stones.

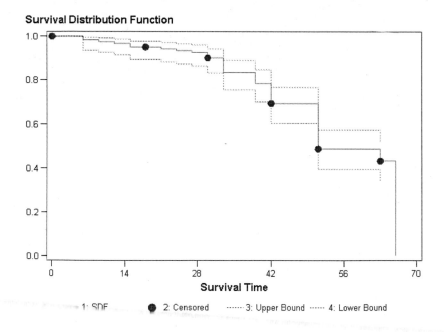

**Fig. 10.10.** Kaplan-Meier survival curve for patients after surgical operation

| Quartile Estimates | | | |
|---|---|---|---|
| | Point | 95% Confidence Interval | |
| Percent | Estimate | [Lower | Upper) |
| 75 | 66.0000 | . | . |
| 50 | 51.0000 | 51.0000 | 66.0000 |
| 25 | 42.0000 | 39.0000 | 51.0000 |

**Fig. 10.11.** Quartile estimates with confidence intervals for patients after surgical operation

It is interesting to compare quartiles in the whole population and subgroups divided by type of treatment. In respect to his analysis the surgery removal of the deposit is more effective than the lithotripsy.

# RECAPITULATION

The set of presented exercises that constitute the further steps in basic statistical analysis represents only a little part of a wide spectrum of statistical analyses. The omitted issues are:

1. **nonlinear analysis regression** – a situation, when the points marked in the coordinates arrangement do not follow the straight line,
2. **logistical regression** – the regression marking the situation approximating the state of probability = 1 or = 0 (the probability of certain feature appearance or its absence).
3. **multidimensional regression** – when one feature's value depends on the values of many other features,
4. **multidimensional** variance analysis (bi-factor or multifactor) – a situation similar to the ANOVA test, taking into account the mean values of two or more features simultaneously.

Moreover, many other methods were not included that are used in medical data analysis and go beyond the traditional statistical methods (procedures not necessarily demanding exact following the schemes presented for statistical tests). An example of such a method is the presented survival analysis.

The handbook objective was approximating the way of reasoning and the principles of drawing detailed conclusions, as well as the method of their generalizing. The theoretical mathematical bases were not penetrated, either, as they can be obtained by the Reader in other handbooks. A very accessible handbook is, published in a beautiful edition: *Wayne W. Daniel: Biostatistics, P297, Seventh Edition, John Wiley & Sons New York, Chichester, Weinheim, Brisbane, Singapore, Toronto, 1999; Klaus Hinkelmann and Oscar Kempthorne: Design and Analysis of Experiments, Revised Edition, Wiley, New York, 1994; Douglas C. Montgomery: Design and Analysis of Experiments. Fourth Edition, Wiley, New York 1997; Jerome L. Myers and Arnold D. Well: Research Design and Statistical Analysis, Earlbaum Associates, Hillsdale, NJ 1995.*

The book "Biostatistics" has already had seven reissues, which is the best testimony of its universal character and popularity. The examples discussed in it are conducted on the basis of SAS packet with the only difference that an older (non-Windows) version of that program was presented.

The Reader will find a sample data base (written in Excel format), designed for self-study data analysis, on the CD that is attached to our handbook. The .xls format enables data importing to any statistical packet accessible to the Reader.

It is worth mentioning that the majority of packets have assumed graphic forms close to Excel dialogue window arrangement. Hence any difficulties in using any statistical packet are rather unlikely.

Analysing the data, one should first of all remember their character. An (incorrect) application of $\chi^2$ test to a measurable variable results in the contingency table construction of large number of columns and rows with very low frequency in each cell (including zero frequency) and provides the entirely incorrect conclusion. This is a very frequent students' mistake. Turning attention to the variable's character (measurable, quantitative) and the qualitative variable (binary in t-Student test) is a condition of the correct test conducting. What is very important, though, if not the most important for the analysis to be successful, is an adequate data preparation. Properly prepared data is a guarantee of the whole analytical procedure correctness.

The Reader finds the courage to conduct independently the analysis of the attached (on CD) data – it means - the handbook achieved its goal. A more advanced analysis conducted by a professional in statistics will be more comprehensible to a medical expert.

**We wish you all the best of luck.**

The data concerning nephrolithiasis whose analysis was presented in the handbook are the demo type data (constructed for the needs of this handbook).

The traffic accidents data on CD were made available by Professor Leszek Brongiel, the Head of the Department of Emergency Medicine and Multiple Trauma of 2nd Chair of General Surgery Collegium Medicum – Jagiellonian University. Author expresses her gratitude for the data that are of vital help in mastering the statistical methods by the students of medical disciplines.

Many thanks to dr Krystyna Dużyk-Żabińska (Chair of Nephrology Collegium Medicum – Jagiellonian University) for professional consultations of urological problems presented in his manual. Without Her help the preparation of this book could be impossible.

# AFTERWORD

In present day reality which is defined as the era of information technology, one should remember of another side of the medical practitioner's work with a specialist in mathematics or information technology, not necessarily limited to the statistical analyses.

Common access to enormous databases and to adequate, often extremely diversified IT instruments opens totally new collaboration possibilities of medical sciences with mathematical applications. The new quality of this collaboration consists in defining common research projects of medical matters in whose realisation an information scientist (a mathematician) can apply non-standard models, verifying the mechanism of processes responsible for the living organisms functioning.

If we run a little ahead and indulge in daydreams, it will prove that solving numerous problems, including the most important one concerning neoplasm forming, becomes possible and even close.

Voices are raised in discussion upon the mechanisms leading to disorders with which organism is unable to cope by itself. There is an audacious hypothesis saying that there are innumerable clinical and experimental data (cells, experimental animals). Most frequently these are very detailed data, concerning the particulars of various processes occurring in the organism both at the stage preceding a neoplasm change and during its expansion. The difficulty in interpretation of those data, sometimes very differentiated consists in the fact, that the tools are missing that would enable examination of a large number of detailed data. Opinions expressed in scientific papers, such as Nature or Science sound that only a close collaboration of mathematicians with physicians will (maybe in nearest future) recognize the correctly functioning mechanisms. The moment the correct processes simulation is possible, it will also be possible to simulate the processes disturbed in the aim-oriented form. It is assumed that it will be possible to simulate a process that reflects what we observe in experiments or clinical practice.

This handbook presents in a short outline the calculating methods of the statistical form. The purpose of this handbook is also to encourage medical students to collaborate with the specialists from mathematics and information technology branches. The most important thing in this collaboration is a common language and mutual confidence in technologies that those disciplines use. If this handbook encourages the Reader to such collaboration, in the same way the purpose for which the handbook has been worked out, will have been reached.

# SUPPLEMENTARY TABLES

**LEVEL OF SIGNIFICANCE**

| NUMBER OF DEGREES OF FREEDOM | 0.99 | 0.98 | 0.95 | 0.90 | 0.80 | 0.70 | 0.50 | 0.30 | 0.20 | 0.10 | 0.05 | 0.02 | 0.01 | 0.001 |
|---|---|---|---|---|---|---|---|---|---|---|---|---|---|---|
| 1 | 0.000 | 0.000 | 0.004 | 0.016 | 0.064 | 0.148 | 0.455 | 1.074 | 1.642 | 2.706 | 3.841 | 5.412 | 6.635 | 10.827 |
| 2 | 0.020 | 0.040 | 0.103 | 0.211 | 0.446 | 0.713 | 1.386 | 2.408 | 3.219 | 4.605 | 5.991 | 7.824 | 9.210 | 13.815 |
| 3 | 0.115 | 0.185 | 0.352 | 0.584 | 1.005 | 1.424 | 2.366 | 3.665 | 4.642 | 6.251 | 7.815 | 9.837 | 11.345 | 16.268 |
| 4 | 0.297 | 0.429 | 0.711 | 1.064 | 1.649 | 2.195 | 3.357 | 4.878 | 5.989 | 7.779 | 9.488 | 11.668 | 13.277 | 18.465 |
| 5 | 0.554 | 0.752 | 1.145 | 1.610 | 2.343 | 3.000 | 4.351 | 6.064 | 7.289 | 9.236 | 11.070 | 13.388 | 15.086 | 20.517 |
| 6 | 0.872 | 1.134 | 1.635 | 2.204 | 3.070 | 3.828 | 5.348 | 7.231 | 8.558 | 10.645 | 12.592 | 15.033 | 16.812 | 22.457 |
| 7 | 1.239 | 1.564 | 2.167 | 2.833 | 3.822 | 4.671 | 6.346 | 8.383 | 9.803 | 12.017 | 14.067 | 16.622 | 18.475 | 24.322 |
| 8 | 1.646 | 2.032 | 2.733 | 3.490 | 4.594 | 5.527 | 7.344 | 9.524 | 11.030 | 13.362 | 15.507 | 18.168 | 20.090 | 26.125 |
| 9 | 2.088 | 2.532 | 3.325 | 4.168 | 5.380 | 6.393 | 8.343 | 10.656 | 12.242 | 14.684 | 16.919 | 19.679 | 21.666 | 27.877 |
| 10 | 2.558 | 3.059 | 3.940 | 4.865 | 6.179 | 7.267 | 9.342 | 11.781 | 13.442 | 15.987 | 18.307 | 21.161 | 23.209 | 29.588 |
| 11 | 3.053 | 3.609 | 4.575 | 5.578 | 6.989 | 8.148 | 10.341 | 12.899 | 14.631 | 17.275 | 19.675 | 22.618 | 24.725 | 31.264 |
| 12 | 3.571 | 4.178 | 5.226 | 6.304 | 7.807 | 9.034 | 11.340 | 14.011 | 15.812 | 18.549 | 21.026 | 24.054 | 26.217 | 32.909 |
| 13 | 4.107 | 4.765 | 5.892 | 7.042 | 8.634 | 9.926 | 12.340 | 15.119 | 16.985 | 19.812 | 22.362 | 25.472 | 27.688 | 34.528 |
| 14 | 4.660 | 5.368 | 6.571 | 7.790 | 9.467 | 10.821 | 13.339 | 16.222 | 18.151 | 21.064 | 23.685 | 26.873 | 29.141 | 36.123 |
| 15 | 5.229 | 5.985 | 7.261 | 8.547 | 10.307 | 11.721 | 14.339 | 17.322 | 19.311 | 22.307 | 24.996 | 28.259 | 30.578 | 37.697 |
| 16 | 5.812 | 6.614 | 7.962 | 9.312 | 11.152 | 12.624 | 15.338 | 18.418 | 20.465 | 23.542 | 26.296 | 29.633 | 32.000 | 39.252 |
| 17 | 6.408 | 7.255 | 8.672 | 10.085 | 12.002 | 13.531 | 16.338 | 19.511 | 21.615 | 24.769 | 27.587 | 30.995 | 33.409 | 40.790 |
| 18 | 7.015 | 7.906 | 9.390 | 10.865 | 12.857 | 14.440 | 17.338 | 20.601 | 22.760 | 25.989 | 28.869 | 32.346 | 34.805 | 42.312 |
| 19 | 7.633 | 8.567 | 10.117 | 11.651 | 13.716 | 15.352 | 18.338 | 21.689 | 23.900 | 27.204 | 30.144 | 33.687 | 36.191 | 43.820 |
| 20 | 8.260 | 9.237 | 10.851 | 12.443 | 14.578 | 16.266 | 19.337 | 22.775 | 25.038 | 28.412 | 31.410 | 35.020 | 37.566 | 45.315 |
| 21 | 8.897 | 9.915 | 11.591 | 13.240 | 15.445 | 17.182 | 20.337 | 23.858 | 26.171 | 29.615 | 32.671 | 36.343 | 38.932 | 46.797 |
| 22 | 9.542 | 10.600 | 12.338 | 14.041 | 16.314 | 18.101 | 21.337 | 24.939 | 27.301 | 30.813 | 33.924 | 37.659 | 40.289 | 48.268 |
| 23 | 10.192 | 11.293 | 13.091 | 14.848 | 17.187 | 19.021 | 22.337 | 26.018 | 28.429 | 32.007 | 35.172 | 38.968 | 41.638 | 49.728 |
| 24 | 10.856 | 11.992 | 13.848 | 15.659 | 18.062 | 19.943 | 23.337 | 27.096 | 29.553 | 33.196 | 36.415 | 40.270 | 42.980 | 51.179 |
| 25 | 11.524 | 12.697 | 14.611 | 16.473 | 18.940 | 20.867 | 24.337 | 28.172 | 30.675 | 34.382 | 37.652 | 41.566 | 44.314 | 52.620 |
| 26 | 12.198 | 13.409 | 15.379 | 17.292 | 19.820 | 21.792 | 25.336 | 29.246 | 31.795 | 35.563 | 38.885 | 42.856 | 45.642 | 54.052 |
| 27 | 12.879 | 14.125 | 16.151 | 18.114 | 20.703 | 22.719 | 26.336 | 30.319 | 32.912 | 36.741 | 40.113 | 44.140 | 46.963 | 55.476 |
| 28 | 13.565 | 14.847 | 16.928 | 18.939 | 21.588 | 23.647 | 27.336 | 31.391 | 34.027 | 37.916 | 41.337 | 45.419 | 48.278 | 56.893 |
| 29 | 14.256 | 15.574 | 17.708 | 19.768 | 22.475 | 24.577 | 28.336 | 32.461 | 35.139 | 39.087 | 42.557 | 46.693 | 49.588 | 58.302 |
| 30 | 14.953 | 16.306 | 18.493 | 20.599 | 23.364 | 25.508 | 29.336 | 33.530 | 36.250 | 40.256 | 43.773 | 47.962 | 50.892 | 59.703 |

**Tab. S.1.** The distribution of the $\chi^2$ test

NUMBER OF DEGREES OF FREEDOM – NUMERATOR

NUMBER OF DEGREES OF FREEDOM – DENOMINATOR

| Denom \ Num | 1 | 2 | 3 | 4 | 5 | 6 | 7 | 8 | 9 | 10 | 12 | 14 | 16 | 18 | 20 |
|---|---|---|---|---|---|---|---|---|---|---|---|---|---|---|---|
| 1 | 161 | 200 | 216 | 225 | 230 | 234 | 237 | 239 | 241 | 242 | 244 | 245 | 246 | 247 | 248 |
| 2 | 18.5 | 19.0 | 19.2 | 19.2 | 19.3 | 19.3 | 19.4 | 19.4 | 19.4 | 19.4 | 19.4 | 19.4 | 19.4 | 19.4 | 19.4 |
| 3 | 10.1 | 9.55 | 9.28 | 9.12 | 9.01 | 8.94 | 8.89 | 8.85 | 8.81 | 8.79 | 8.74 | 8.74 | 8.69 | 8.67 | 8.66 |
| 4 | 7.71 | 6.94 | 6.59 | 6.39 | 6.26 | 6.16 | 6.09 | 6.04 | 6.00 | 5.96 | 5.91 | 5.91 | 5.84 | 5.82 | 5.80 |
| 5 | 6.61 | 5.79 | 5.41 | 5.19 | 5.05 | 4.95 | 4.88 | 4.82 | 4.77 | 4.74 | 4.68 | 4.68 | 4.60 | 4.58 | 4.56 |
| 6 | 5.99 | 5.14 | 4.76 | 4.53 | 4.39 | 4.28 | 4.21 | 4.15 | 4.10 | 4.06 | 4.00 | 4.00 | 3.92 | 3.90 | 3.87 |
| 7 | 5.59 | 4.74 | 4.35 | 4.12 | 3.97 | 3.87 | 3.79 | 3.73 | 3.68 | 3.64 | 3.57 | 3.57 | 3.49 | 3.47 | 3.44 |
| 8 | 5.32 | 4.46 | 4.07 | 3.84 | 3.69 | 3.58 | 3.50 | 3.44 | 3.39 | 3.35 | 3.28 | 3.28 | 3.20 | 3.17 | 3.15 |
| 9 | 5.12 | 4.26 | 3.86 | 3.63 | 3.48 | 3.37 | 3.29 | 3.23 | 3.18 | 3.14 | 3.07 | 3.07 | 2.99 | 2.96 | 2.94 |
| 10 | 4.96 | 4.10 | 3.71 | 3.48 | 3.33 | 3.22 | 3.14 | 3.07 | 3.02 | 2.98 | 2.91 | 2.91 | 2.83 | 2.80 | 2.77 |
| 11 | 4.84 | 3.98 | 3.59 | 3.36 | 3.20 | 3.09 | 3.01 | 2.95 | 2.90 | 2.85 | 2.79 | 2.79 | 2.70 | 2.67 | 2.65 |
| 12 | 4.75 | 3.89 | 3.49 | 3.26 | 3.11 | 3.00 | 2.91 | 2.85 | 2.80 | 2.75 | 2.69 | 2.69 | 2.60 | 2.57 | 2.54 |
| 13 | 4.67 | 3.81 | 3.41 | 3.18 | 3.03 | 2.92 | 2.83 | 2.77 | 2.71 | 2.67 | 2.60 | 2.60 | 2.51 | 2.48 | 2.46 |
| 14 | 4.60 | 3.74 | 3.34 | 3.11 | 2.96 | 2.85 | 2.76 | 2.70 | 2.65 | 2.60 | 2.53 | 2.53 | 2.44 | 2.41 | 2.39 |
| 15 | 4.54 | 3.68 | 3.29 | 3.06 | 2.90 | 2.79 | 2.71 | 2.64 | 2.59 | 2.54 | 2.48 | 2.48 | 2.38 | 2.35 | 2.33 |
| 16 | 4.49 | 3.63 | 3.24 | 3.01 | 2.85 | 2.74 | 2.66 | 2.59 | 2.54 | 2.49 | 2.42 | 2.42 | 2.33 | 2.30 | 2.28 |
| 17 | 4.45 | 3.59 | 3.20 | 2.96 | 2.81 | 2.70 | 2.61 | 2.55 | 2.49 | 2.45 | 2.38 | 2.38 | 2.29 | 2.26 | 2.23 |
| 18 | 4.41 | 3.55 | 3.16 | 2.93 | 2.77 | 2.66 | 2.58 | 2.51 | 2.46 | 2.41 | 2.34 | 2.34 | 2.25 | 2.22 | 2.19 |
| 19 | 4.38 | 3.52 | 3.13 | 2.90 | 2.74 | 2.63 | 2.54 | 2.48 | 2.42 | 2.38 | 2.31 | 2.31 | 2.21 | 2.18 | 2.16 |
| 20 | 4.35 | 3.49 | 3.10 | 2.87 | 2.71 | 2.60 | 2.51 | 2.45 | 2.39 | 2.35 | 2.28 | 2.28 | 2.18 | 2.15 | 2.12 |
| 21 | 4.32 | 3.47 | 3.07 | 2.84 | 2.68 | 2.57 | 2.49 | 2.42 | 2.37 | 2.32 | 2.25 | 2.25 | 2.16 | 2.12 | 2.10 |
| 22 | 4.30 | 3.44 | 3.05 | 2.82 | 2.66 | 2.55 | 2.46 | 2.40 | 2.34 | 2.30 | 2.23 | 2.23 | 2.13 | 2.10 | 2.07 |
| 23 | 4.28 | 3.42 | 3.03 | 2.80 | 2.64 | 2.53 | 2.44 | 2.37 | 2.32 | 2.27 | 2.20 | 2.20 | 2.11 | 2.07 | 2.05 |
| 24 | 4.26 | 3.40 | 3.01 | 2.78 | 2.62 | 2.51 | 2.42 | 2.36 | 2.30 | 2.25 | 2.18 | 2.18 | 2.09 | 2.05 | 2.03 |
| 25 | 4.24 | 3.39 | 2.99 | 2.76 | 2.60 | 2.49 | 2.40 | 2.34 | 2.28 | 2.24 | 2.16 | 2.16 | 2.07 | 2.04 | 2.01 |

**Tab. S.2.** The distribution of the F-Snedecor test for the significance level 5%

NUMBER OF DEGREES OF FREEDOM — NUMERATOR

| Denom. \ Num. | 22 | 24 | 26 | 28 | 30 | 35 | 40 | 45 | 50 | 60 | 80 | 100 | 200 | 500 | ∞ |
|---|---|---|---|---|---|---|---|---|---|---|---|---|---|---|---|
| 26 | 1.97 | 1.95 | 1.93 | 1.91 | 1.90 | 1.87 | 1.85 | 1.84 | 1.82 | 1.80 | 1.78 | 1.76 | 1.73 | 1.71 | 1.69 |
| 27 | 1.95 | 1.93 | 1.91 | 1.90 | 1.88 | 1.86 | 1.84 | 1.82 | 1.81 | 1.79 | 1.76 | 1.74 | 1.71 | 1.69 | 1.67 |
| 28 | 1.93 | 1.91 | 1.90 | 1.88 | 1.87 | 1.84 | 1.82 | 1.80 | 1.79 | 1.77 | 1.74 | 1.73 | 1.69 | 1.67 | 1.65 |
| 29 | 1.92 | 1.90 | 1.88 | 1.87 | 1.85 | 1.83 | 1.81 | 1.79 | 1.77 | 1.75 | 1.73 | 1.71 | 1.67 | 1.65 | 1.64 |
| 30 | 1.91 | 1.89 | 1.87 | 1.85 | 1.84 | 1.81 | 1.79 | 1.77 | 1.76 | 1.74 | 1.71 | 1.70 | 1.66 | 1.64 | 1.62 |
| 32 | 1.88 | 1.86 | 1.85 | 1.83 | 1.82 | 1.79 | 1.77 | 1.75 | 1.74 | 1.71 | 1.69 | 1.67 | 1.63 | 1.61 | 1.59 |
| 34 | 1.86 | 1.84 | 1.82 | 1.80 | 1.80 | 1.77 | 1.75 | 1.73 | 1.71 | 1.69 | 1.66 | 1.65 | 1.61 | 1.59 | 1.57 |
| 36 | 1.85 | 1.82 | 1.81 | 1.79 | 1.78 | 1.75 | 1.73 | 1.71 | 1.69 | 1.67 | 1.64 | 1.62 | 1.59 | 1.56 | 1.55 |
| 38 | 1.83 | 1.81 | 1.79 | 1.77 | 1.76 | 1.73 | 1.71 | 1.69 | 1.68 | 1.65 | 1.62 | 1.61 | 1.57 | 1.54 | 1.53 |
| 40 | 1.81 | 1.79 | 1.77 | 1.76 | 1.74 | 1.72 | 1.69 | 1.67 | 1.66 | 1.64 | 1.61 | 1.59 | 1.55 | 1.53 | 1.51 |
| 42 | 1.80 | 1.78 | 1.76 | 1.74 | 1.73 | 1.70 | 1.68 | 1.66 | 1.65 | 1.62 | 1.59 | 1.57 | 1.53 | 1.51 | 1.49 |
| 44 | 1.79 | 1.77 | 1.75 | 1.73 | 1.72 | 1.69 | 1.67 | 1.65 | 1.63 | 1.61 | 1.58 | 1.56 | 1.52 | 1.49 | 1.48 |
| 46 | 1.78 | 1.76 | 1.74 | 1.72 | 1.71 | 1.68 | 1.65 | 1.64 | 1.62 | 1.60 | 1.57 | 1.55 | 1.51 | 1.48 | 1.46 |
| 48 | 1.77 | 1.75 | 1.73 | 1.72 | 1.70 | 1.67 | 1.64 | 1.62 | 1.61 | 1.59 | 1.56 | 1.54 | 1.49 | 1.47 | 1.45 |
| 50 | 1.76 | 1.74 | 1.72 | 1.70 | 1.69 | 1.66 | 1.63 | 1.61 | 1.60 | 1.58 | 1.54 | 1.52 | 1.48 | 1.46 | 1.44 |
| 60 | 1.72 | 1.70 | 1.68 | 1.66 | 1.65 | 1.62 | 1.59 | 1.57 | 1.56 | 1.53 | 1.50 | 1.48 | 1.44 | 1.41 | 1.39 |
| 80 | 1.68 | 1.65 | 1.63 | 1.62 | 1.60 | 1.57 | 1.54 | 1.52 | 1.51 | 1.48 | 1.45 | 1.43 | 1.38 | 1.35 | 1.32 |
| 100 | 1.65 | 1.63 | 1.61 | 1.59 | 1.57 | 1.54 | 1.52 | 1.49 | 1.48 | 1.45 | 1.41 | 1.39 | 1.34 | 1.31 | 1.28 |
| 125 | 1.63 | 1.60 | 1.58 | 1.57 | 1.55 | 1.52 | 1.49 | 1.47 | 1.45 | 1.42 | 1.39 | 1.36 | 1.31 | 1.27 | 1.25 |
| 150 | 1.61 | 1.59 | 1.57 | 1.55 | 1.53 | 1.50 | 1.48 | 1.45 | 1.44 | 1.41 | 1.37 | 1.34 | 1.29 | 1.25 | 1.22 |
| 200 | 1.60 | 1.57 | 1.55 | 1.53 | 1.52 | 1.48 | 1.46 | 1.43 | 1.41 | 1.39 | 1.35 | 1.32 | 1.26 | 1.22 | 1.19 |
| 300 | 1.58 | 1.55 | 1.53 | 1.51 | 1.50 | 1.46 | 1.43 | 1.41 | 1.39 | 1.36 | 1.32 | 1.30 | 1.23 | 1.19 | 1.15 |
| 500 | 1.56 | 1.54 | 1.52 | 1.50 | 1.48 | 1.45 | 1.42 | 1.40 | 1.38 | 1.34 | 1.30 | 1.28 | 1.21 | 1.16 | 1.11 |
| 1000 | 1.55 | 1.53 | 1.51 | 1.49 | 1.47 | 1.44 | 1.41 | 1.38 | 1.36 | 1.33 | 1.29 | 1.26 | 1.19 | 1.13 | 1.08 |
| ∞ | 1.54 | 1.52 | 1.50 | 1.48 | 1.46 | 1.42 | 1.39 | 1.37 | 1.35 | 1.32 | 1.27 | 1.24 | 1.17 | 1.11 | 1.00 |

NUMBER OF DEGREES OF FREEDOM — DENOMINATOR

cont. **Tab. S.2.** The distribution of the F-Snedecor test for the significance level 5%

NUMBER OF DEGREES OF FREEDOM

LEVEL OF SIGNIFICANCE

| NUMBER OF DEGREES OF FREEDOM | 0.001 | 0.01 | 0.02 | 0.05 | 0.1 | 0.2 | 0.3 | 0.4 | 0.5 | 0.6 | 0.7 | 0.8 | 0.9 |
|---|---|---|---|---|---|---|---|---|---|---|---|---|---|
| 1 | 636.62 | 63.657 | 31.821 | 12.706 | 6.315 | 3.078 | 1.963 | 1.376 | 1.000 | 0.727 | 0.510 | 0.325 | 0.158 |
| 2 | 31.598 | 6.925 | 6.965 | 4.303 | 2.920 | 1.886 | 1.386 | 1.061 | 0.816 | 0.617 | 0.445 | 0.289 | 0.142 |
| 3 | 12.941 | 5.841 | 4.541 | 3.182 | 2.353 | 1.638 | 1.250 | 0.978 | 0.765 | 0.584 | 0.424 | 0.277 | 0.137 |
| 4 | 8.610 | 4.604 | 3.747 | 2.776 | 2.132 | 1.533 | 1.190 | 0.941 | 0.741 | 0.569 | 0.414 | 0.271 | 0.134 |
| 5 | 6.859 | 4.032 | 3.365 | 2.571 | 2.015 | 1.476 | 1.156 | 0.920 | 0.727 | 0.559 | 0.408 | 0.267 | 0.132 |
| 6 | 5.959 | 3.707 | 3.143 | 2.447 | 1.943 | 1.440 | 1.134 | 0.906 | 0.718 | 0.553 | 0.404 | 0.265 | 0.131 |
| 7 | 5.405 | 3.499 | 2.998 | 2.365 | 1.895 | 1.415 | 1.119 | 0.896 | 0.711 | 0.549 | 0.402 | 0.263 | 0.130 |
| 8 | 5.041 | 3.355 | 2.896 | 2.306 | 1.860 | 1.397 | 1.108 | 0.889 | 0.706 | 0.546 | 0.399 | 0.262 | 0.130 |
| 9 | 4.781 | 3.250 | 2.821 | 2.262 | 1.833 | 1.383 | 1.100 | 0.883 | 0.703 | 0.543 | 0.398 | 0.261 | 0.129 |
| 10 | 4.587 | 3.169 | 2.764 | 2.228 | 1.812 | 1.372 | 1.093 | 0.879 | 0.700 | 0.542 | 0.397 | 0.260 | 0.129 |
| 11 | 4.437 | 3.106 | 2.718 | 2.201 | 1.796 | 1.363 | 1.088 | 0.876 | 0.697 | 0.540 | 0.396 | 0.260 | 0.129 |
| 12 | 4.318 | 3.055 | 2.681 | 2.179 | 1.782 | 1.356 | 1.083 | 0.873 | 0.695 | 0.539 | 0.395 | 0.259 | 0.128 |
| 13 | 4.221 | 3.012 | 2.650 | 2.160 | 1.771 | 1.350 | 1.079 | 0.870 | 0.694 | 0.538 | 0.394 | 0.259 | 0.128 |
| 14 | 4.140 | 2.977 | 2.624 | 2.145 | 1.761 | 1.345 | 1.076 | 0.868 | 0.692 | 0.537 | 0.393 | 0.258 | 0.128 |
| 15 | 4.073 | 2.947 | 2.602 | 2.131 | 1.753 | 1.341 | 1.074 | 0.866 | 0.691 | 0.536 | 0.393 | 0.258 | 0.128 |
| 16 | 4.015 | 2.921 | 2.583 | 2.120 | 1.746 | 1.337 | 1.337 | 0.865 | 0.690 | 0.535 | 0.392 | 0.258 | 0.128 |
| 17 | 3.965 | 2.898 | 2.567 | 2.110 | 1.740 | 1.333 | 1.333 | 0.863 | 0.689 | 0.534 | 0.392 | 0.257 | 0.128 |
| 18 | 3.922 | 2.878 | 2.552 | 2.101 | 1.734 | 1.330 | 1.330 | 0.862 | 0.688 | 0.534 | 0.392 | 0.257 | 0.127 |
| 19 | 3.883 | 2.861 | 2.539 | 2.093 | 1.729 | 1.328 | 1.328 | 0.861 | 0.688 | 0.533 | 0.391 | 0.257 | 0.127 |
| 20 | 3.850 | 2.845 | 2.528 | 2.086 | 1.725 | 1.325 | 1.325 | 0.860 | 0.687 | 0.533 | 0.391 | 0.257 | 0.127 |
| 21 | 3.819 | 2.831 | 2.518 | 2.080 | 1.721 | 1.323 | 1.323 | 0.859 | 0.686 | 0.532 | 0.391 | 0.257 | 0.127 |
| 22 | 3.792 | 2.819 | 2.508 | 2.074 | 1.717 | 1.321 | 1.321 | 0.858 | 0.686 | 0.532 | 0.390 | 0.256 | 0.127 |
| 23 | 3.767 | 2.809 | 2.500 | 2.069 | 1.714 | 1.319 | 1.319 | 0.858 | 0.685 | 0.532 | 0.390 | 0.256 | 0.127 |
| 24 | 3.745 | 2.797 | 2.492 | 2.064 | 1.711 | 1.318 | 1.318 | 0.857 | 0.685 | 0.531 | 0.390 | 0.256 | 0.127 |
| 25 | 3.725 | 2.787 | 2.485 | 2.060 | 1.708 | 1.316 | 1.316 | 0.856 | 0.684 | 0.531 | 0.390 | 0.256 | 0.127 |
| 26 | 3.707 | 2.779 | 2.479 | 2.056 | 1.706 | 1.315 | 1.315 | 0.856 | 0.684 | 0.531 | 0.390 | 0.256 | 0.127 |
| 27 | 3.690 | 2.771 | 2.473 | 2.052 | 1.703 | 1.314 | 1.314 | 0.855 | 0.684 | 0.531 | 0.389 | 0.256 | 0.127 |
| 28 | 3.674 | 2.763 | 2.467 | 2.048 | 1.701 | 1.313 | 1.313 | 0.855 | 0.683 | 0.530 | 0.389 | 0.256 | 0.127 |
| 29 | 3.659 | 2.756 | 2.462 | 2.045 | 1.699 | 1.311 | 1.311 | 0.854 | 0.683 | 0.530 | 0.389 | 0.256 | 0.127 |
| 30 | 3.646 | 2.750 | 2.457 | 2.042 | 1.697 | 1.310 | 1.310 | 0.854 | 0.683 | 0.530 | 0.389 | 0.256 | 0.127 |
| 40 | 3.551 | 2.704 | 2.423 | 2.021 | 1.684 | 1.303 | 1.303 | 0.851 | 0.681 | 0.529 | 0.388 | 0.255 | 0.126 |
| 60 | 3.460 | 2.660 | 2.390 | 2.000 | 1.671 | 1.296 | 1.296 | 0.848 | 0.679 | 0.527 | 0.387 | 0.254 | 0.126 |
| 120 | 3.373 | 2.617 | 2.358 | 1.980 | 1.658 | 1.289 | 1.289 | 0.845 | 0.677 | 0.526 | 0.386 | 0.254 | 0.126 |
| ∞ | 3.291 | 2.576 | 2.326 | 1.96 | 1.645 | 1.282 | 1.282 | 0.842 | 0.674 | 0.524 | 0.385 | 0.253 | 0.126 |

NUMBER OF DEGREES OF FREEDOM

**Tab. S.3.** The distribution of the t-Student test

# VOCABULARY

## A

**Additivity rule in the probability calculus** – the probability of the occurrence of two or more mutually exclusive events is equal to the sum of their individual probabilities.

**Alternative hypothesis** – the hypothesis (called $H_1$ or $H_a$) expressing the contradiction to the null hypothesis $H_0$. If the null hypothesis appears to be rejected, the alternative hypothesis is believed to be true. *See* null hypothesis.

**Analysis of variance** – a statistical technique for determining whether exists difference between groups specified due to a classification factors.

**ANOVA test** – the test for a common mean in multiple groups. Extension of T-test which is limited to the comparison of only two groups. ANOVA assumes that all the samples have the common origin (belong to the same population) (null hypothesis) with the alternative hypothesis that some of them (or even one of them) differ significantly versus the others. The relation between "within" variation (the internal distributions in groups) in relation to "between" (distribution of mean values representing each group) is calculated and assessed as significant. The test expects the distribution of the variable under consideration is of the normal character in each group. *See* F-test, Bonferroni test.

**Arithmetic mean** – the sum of all numbers divide by the number of items in the list, it represent the measurement of central tendency, it is the value around which all other values expressing particular variable are concentrated.

## B

**Bar charts** – the graphical display of data classified into categories (qualitative variable – for example – day of the week). Resented by rectangular bars of the height proportional to the percentage (or absolute number) of the events under consideration taking place on the particular day (for example the number of patients transported to emergency department with the alcohol present in their blood).

**Bimodal distribution** – the continuous probability distribution with two modes, what is visualized as two peaks (local maxima) distribution. It suggests that the data which arise from two distinct populations (the distribution of blood pressure of people addicted to coffee and those who are not).

**Biostatistics** – statistics applied specifically to medical and biological disciplines including practical medicine as well as agriculture developing specific techniques adequate for the medical problems. *See* – for example – survival analysis.

**Bonferroni test** – the *post hoc* test determining the significant differences between group means in an analysis of variance.

**Box-and-whisker plot** – the graphical display to highlighting important features of a variable. Box (localized on the axis representing the variable under consideration) size represents usually the minimum value, the lower quartile, the median, the upper quartile and maximum in the sample. Each parameter is in differentiated graphical form (short lines, small boxes, parentheses, etc.). The relative positions of these parameters visualize for example the skewness of the distribution. *See* skewness.

# C

**Censored observation** – partially observed information about the time of the event under consideration. The exact time of the event is unknown as it may not yet have occurred or be known to have occurred. For example, in a study of time recurrence of a particular medical condition, some patients may not experience a recurrence at the end of the study, some may drop out or the contact with them may be lost to follow-up, some may experience the event of interest during successive medical visits and the others may pass away due to other reasons than the one under consideration. Censoring may be of right censoring form – the end event of the subject's follow-up is not observed; or left censoring – the starting point of the event is not noticeable (unrecognized appearance of the disease).

**Central tendency** – *See* measures of location.

**Chi-square test** – the statistical significance test to verify the hypotheses of categorical data and their distributions in particular. The elements of the sample collected in contingency tables (each cell of the table represents frequency of the one – row and second – column – representing the observed combination of two non-measurable variables).

**Class interval** – definition of intervals allowing construction of histogram. *See* histogram.

**Confidence interval** – a range of values calculated from the sample for a parameter being estimated on a specified level of confidence. A 95% confidence interval is defined in such a way that the probability of the fact that real value of the estimated parameter is outside the interval is equal to 5% (0.05).

**Contingency table** – cross-tabulation that arises when a sample from some population is classified with respect to two or more quantitative variables.

**Continuous variable** – the variable with no exclusions of values in the reasonable interval. For example somebody's height: there is no exclusion in the interval between 100 cm and 250 cm. Any real value from this range may express somebody's height. *See* discrete variable.

**Correlation** – the tendency of the relationship between values of two random variables to increase or decrease in consistent or inconsistent way.

**Correlation coefficient** – the quantitative measurements of the strength of the mutual relationship between two variables. The maximum value of the cc is +1.0., when the points all lie exactly on a straight line and the variables are positively correlated (the increase of the value of one of them results as increase of the value of the second one). The minimum value equals to -1.0., when the points all lie exactly on the straight line and the variables are negatively correlated (the increase of the value of one of them results as decrease of the value of the second one). No correlation is observed when cc is equal to 0.0. The significance of the cc may be estimated using the test assessing its value as significant or not.

**Critical region** – the rejection region for $p < \alpha$.

**Critical value** – the values of the test statistics that separate the rejection and non-rejection regions.

**Cumulative probability** – the sum of probabilities (frequencies) for variables of values below the defined one – for example $X_c$.

# D

**Data collection** – the process to put observations into electronic format for computer analysis. The accurate and collection of data is crucial for statistical analysis. The correct data – the correct conclusions driven from them. Two kinds of possible errors: mistaken data introduced, missing information. The unified units for measurements must be defined before the database initiation. The clerical error may be easily eliminated by electronic tools applied for the data base organization (program checks the number of obligatory digits, the upper and lower limits of reasonable values, etc.). The discussion of the medical researcher with the specialist preparing electronic tool may give additional limitations specific for particular database (data base) (particular variable) verifying its correctness.

**Monitoring** – the role of the administrator of the database. It includes permanent analysis of the database correctness and hardware-software cooperation.

**Safety** – the confidential character of medical data requires protection of data base and restrictions in access to the data. The limited access to the data base (administrator, the person-in-charge, users, patients etc.) makes the control of accessibility easy. The tools protecting the database against the hackers are necessary.

**Management** – the systematic management of large scale database. The compatibility with different statistical packages is highly expected. The applicability of the data for Excel package seems to be important for users interested in permanent monitoring of data collected.

**Analysis** – the applicability of all possible statistical methods to describe data and to recognize the relations, dependences and differences between sub-groups discriminated according to defined criteria.

**Mining in medicine** – the discipline linking the computer science with statistics oriented on extracting useful knowledge from databases. The search for association, relations, classification rules between collected variables which may influence the field of detailed research particularly in the case of rare or still unrecognized medical phenomena (new diseases, neglected disease, etc.).

**Data – graphic presentation** – *See* bar chart, pie-chart.

**Data – types of** – *See* variables.

**Decision rule** – the rule defining the conditions to reject $H_0$ if the computed value of the test statistics falls in the rejection region and to fail to reject $H_0$ if it falls in the non-rejection region.

**Degrees of freedom** – an exclusive concept that occurs throughout statistics. ($df$) means the number of independent units of information in a sample relevant to the estimation of parameter or the calculation of a statistics.

**Density function of probability** – a function that represents a probability distribution in terms of integrals

**Descriptive analysis** – *See* descriptive statistics.

**Descriptive statistics** – summaries designed to encapsulate meaningful aspects of dataset – there are three basic techniques: graphical display, tabular description, summary statistics.

**Discontinuous variable** – there are exclusions in the reasonable range of values for all possible values of the particular variable forms a finite or countable infinite set. For example: number of patients in the hospital. Only natural numbers are possible to express this variable. For example: the value 32.74 is a priori excluded.

**Discrete variable** – *See* discontinuous variable.

**Dispersion** – the distribution of values in relation to mean value. *See* range, standard deviation, variance.

**Distribution free procedures** – *See* nonparametric tests.

**Distribution normal** – *See* normal distribution.

# E

**Empirical distribution** – the characteristics of particular variable in form of the frequency of the occurrence of the values belonging to particular ranges of this variable received according to the sample data collection. *See* histogram.

**Errors in hypothesis tests** – the error committed when the true null hypothesis is rejected or when a false null hypothesis is not rejected. *See* the type I error and type II error.

**Estimation** – part of statistical inference together with hypothesis testing. The process entails calculating (from the data of the sample) some statistics that is assumed as an approximation of the corresponding parameters of the population from which the sample was drawn. *See* hypothesis testing.

**Evidence based medicine** – the summary of medical experiences in medical health care to make available the assessment and applying relevant evidence for better healthcare decision-makings linking multi-disciplinary specializations, like genetics, immunology, epidemiology, etc., with the medical practice.

**Extreme values** – the largest and the smallest values as they appear in the sample. *See* range.

# F

**False positive** – the indication of a positive status as while the true status which is negative.

**False negative** – the indication of the negative status when the true status is positive.

**F-distribution** – the continuous probability distribution (also known as Snedecor's F distribution) used mainly in the analysis of variance (F-test).

**Frequency table** – *See* contingency table.

**F-test** – the procedure allowing verification of the significance of the difference between variances as they appear in two (or more – *See* ANOVA test) compared group.

# G

**Gaussian distribution** – probability distribution accordant to the Gaussian function.

**Gaussian function** – the function of exponential form $f(x) = ae^{\frac{(x-b)^2}{2c^2}}$ the graphic presentation of which is the symmetric bell-shaped line.

**Goodness-of-fit test** – nonparametric test comparing the experimentally observed distribution with the theoretical one (normal one in particular) and classifying the difference as negligibly small (null hypothesis) or significant (alternative hypothesis).

**Graphical representation** – *See* histogram, scatter-plot, box-and-whisker plot.

**Grouped data** – data grouped according to the qualitative or quantitative (defined range of values) criteria. Particularly necessary for the preparation of histogram.

# H

**Histogram** – the graphical presentation of the frequencies of values belonging to defined ranges of values. Each range is represented by a vertical bar of the height is proportional to the frequency of particular interval. The base of each bar is of size of the size of interval. The histogram is aimed to show the distribution of particular values classified according to defined intervals.

**Hypothesis**

**Alternative** – *See* alternative hypothesis,

**Decision rule** – decision concerning the rejection or non-rejection of null hypothesis depending on the value of statistics falls or not in the rejection region,

**Null** – *See* null hypothesis.

**Hypothesis verification** – the procedure to test the hypotheses expressed in null hypothesis versus the alternative hypothesis. The decision of choosing one of competing hypotheses (null and alternative) depends on the level of significance and number of degrees of freedom, which is defined specifically for each test.

# I

**Independent events** – two events are independent when one of them occurred has no effect on the probability of the occurrence of the second one.

**Independence test** – the non-parametric $\chi^2$ test for independence is applied to assess whether the two variables (in one single group) represent the same distribution of subjects across categories in one variable is the same for the categories of the other variable.

**Inferential statistics** – the set of procedures by which we reach a conclusion about a population on the basis of the information contained in a sample drawn from that population.

**Intercept** – the parameter present in the linear function expressing the value of $Y$ for $x = 0$.

**Interval** – the range of values expressing the upper and lower limit of the data set or for the class; *See* – histogram.

# K

**Kaplan-Meier estimator** – the method to estimate the survival function (survival curve expressing the percentage of the patients surviving particular period of time – in relative scale starting at point 0 when the medical event under consideration took place). It expresses the conditional probability to survive up to the certain time taking into account the probability to survive the preceding time periods.

**Kaplan-Meier plot** – the graphical presentation of the probability changes as depending on time. The time = 0 (starting point) is described by probability = 1.0 (all patients alive). The curve approaches gradually the $X$-axis (time axis) proportionally to the number of patients surviving sequential time periods. Usually 5 years time period is treated as survival. The probability level reached for 5 years interval approximately estimates the mortality characteristic for the disease under consideration. One must emphasize that such curve shows only the pattern of mortality and can be used only as the general tendency which in particular case may appear as inaccurate.

**Kolmogorov-Smirnov test** – the non-parametric test estimating the goodness-of-fit. The null hypothesis expresses neglecting the difference between the theoretical distribution (in particular the normal distribution) and the experimentally observed one. *See* also – $\chi^2$ test of goodness-of-fit.

**Kruskal-Wallis test** – The non-parametric test to compare more than two groups (extension of Mann-Whitney test) on the basis of sum of rank comparison.

**Kurtosis** – the term expressing the character of the peak shape in probability distribution. The sharper peak, the higher kurtosis, the slow decrease of values versus the highest one – the lower kurtosis.

# L

**Least squares estimation** – the general model to estimate the parameters of regression function (the linear regression in particular). The values of parameters (slope and intercept) are calculated to minimize the sum of squares distances between observed and expected outcomes. Both parameters to be treated as representing particular scatter plot distribution may be estimated applying special test for significance of the parameter under consideration.

**Limitation** – some tests do not accept low number of observations. The number of observation must be larger than 5 in each cell of the contingency table to apply the chi-square test.

**Linear regression** – the technique to characterize quantitatively the relation between the variable "$y$" assumed to be the outcome of the particular value (independent variable) of the value "$x$" assumed to express the origin of the observed "$y$" variable (dependent variable). The parameters of linear function (slope and intercept) can be calculated applying the least squares method. Their significance may be estimated applying appropriate test of significance.

**Linear regression function** – the function of the form $y = a\,x + b$ which represents the relationship between independent and dependent variables. *See* slope and intercept.

# M

**Mann-Whitney rank sum test** – The non-parametric test (known also as Wilcoxon rank sum test) applied to estimate the significance between two samples testing the differences in shape and spread of the data in two compared groups.

**Mean** – the measure of location expressing a typical value of the set of observations of measurable (continuous as well as discrete) character. It is calculated as sum of all elements divided by the number of elements. The mean value is referred to population – $\mu$ (its value is unknown due to unknown number of elements in population) and sample – $\bar{x}$ (known value – known number of elements belonging to the sample).

**Measure of spread** – *See* variability.

**Measures of spread** – the measure to what extend the values are scattered around their typical value which is the mean value. The parameters expressing this characteristics are: range, variance and standard deviation.

**Measurable variable** – assignment of real value to object or event according to a set of rules (for example – units for particular measurement).

**Measurements of location** – mean, median, mode. *See* central tendency.

**Median** – one of the methods to express the measure of location (or central tendency) expressed by the middle value in the ordered observations set. It may be called as "halfway" value. For odd number of elements, the median is the central one, for even number of elements the mean value of the two central values.

**Medical statistics** – the discipline of science oriented on collecting, analyzing and interpreting medical data. The medical statistics especially applied for medical data describing the diseases, health, healthcare, etc. The descriptive statistics – calculation of parameters describing particular data set (central tendency, dispersion, distribution, etc.).

**Missing data** – The well-prepared statistical studies draw a representative sample from the population according to preliminary prepared plan and protocol. Despite the preparations some data are unavailable or absent. Missing data cannot be completed in any ways due to their individuality and specificity.

**Mode** – the measure of location expressed by the most frequently occurring value of the variable under consideration. If more than one value appears with the same high frequency, the two or more values are treated as modes (two-, three-modal set).

# N

**Non-linear regression function** – the function representing the set of points of other than linear form.

**Non-parametric methods** – the tests applied to the data of qualitative character or to the measurable variables the distribution of which appeared to be different than normal. Non-parametric tests expect some special conditions to be satisfied. They are oriented on the analysis of contingency tables (qualitative variables), goodness-of-fit tests, the tests based on ranks to estimate the significance between the groups (two or more).

**Normal distribution (Gaussian distribution)** – the family of continuous probability distributions of symmetric, unimodal, bell-shaped curve expressed by the Gaussian function with two parameters (location and scale): mean value μ and variance (σ – standard deviation squared). The standard normal distribution is the normal distribution with a mean equal to zero and a variance equal to one.

**Null hypothesis** – the hypothesis being tested (called $H_0$) expressing the statement concerning the population. It usually takes the form neglecting existence of any difference or association. *See* alternative hypothesis.

# O

**One-sided test** – the alternative hypothesis states that the difference (between two mean values for example) is significant. The direction of the one-sided-test is directional – it means that the one is significantly larger ($\bar{x}_A \rangle \bar{x}_B$) or significantly lower ($\bar{x}_A \langle \bar{x}_B$). *See* two-sided-test.

**Ordered data set** – the randomly (or chronologically) collected data put in increasing or decreasing order

# P

**Parameter** – a descriptive measure defines a quantity of certain characteristics computed from observed data.

**Parametric test** – the statistical procedure concerning the estimation of parameters describing probability distribution or testing hypotheses about these parameters

**Patients characteristics** – *See* questionnaire.

**Pearson's correlation coefficient** – the most widely used measure of association between two variables of linear relation, it describes the strength of dependence in range from –1 to +1.

**Percentile** – is the value of some variable below which a certain percent of observations fall

**Pie-chart** – the graphical presentation of frequencies or percentages in form of the circular graph divide into sectors proportionally to the observed values. Due to criticism (no visualization of the sample size, misleading use of 3-dimensionality, dependence on the rotational orientation of particular slices) used mostly for advertising and easy visualization techniques. Table presentation of data is preferable for scientific purposes.

**Pilot studies** – small-scale experiments preceding the full-scale analysis – partial data collection to get the general information about the population under consideration. The pilot study improves the main research suggesting the sample size, equilibration of the information (balance between sources and consequences, etc.).

**Population** – the entire collection of entities satisfying defined conditions.

**Post-hoc analysis** – in English "after the event" – analysis performed after preceding performance of the test. *See* Bonferroni test.

**Power of the test** – the control of the error type II designated as $1 - \beta$ expressing the probability to reject a false null hypothesis. *See* error type I and error type II.

**Probability** – two connotations: mathematical discipline of the study of uncertainty and numerical scale [0;1] to specify the likelihood or chance that something will happen. The second approach is presented mostly in the manual under consideration due to bright knowledge of mathematics which is necessary to investigate the theory of probability.

**Probability calculation** – the classical definition says, that the relation of N expressing number of events called success to all possible events (together success and non-success) M is equal to N/M.

**Probability density function** – *See* Density function.

**Probability distribution** – identifies either the probability of each value of a variable (when the variable is discrete) or the probability of the fact that value falls into the specific interval (continuous variable).

**Probability plot** – graphical technique for estimate whether data forms certain distribution, data are plotted against a theoretical distribution in such a way that points should form a straight line when distributions are compliant *See* also histogram.

**Problem definition** – The subject of medical research requires preparation to be applicable to the statistical methodology what means that the population, sample generation, set of data (structure of the information record) shall be defined.

**p-value** – level to assess the reliability of null hypothesis. The p-value measures the probability to be mistaken to accept the null hypothesis to be true.

# Q

**Qualitative variable** – *See* variable qualitative.

**Quartile** – first is equal the 25-percentile, second is equal the 50-percentile, third is equal the 75-percentile. *See* percentile.

**Questionnaire(s)** – a pattern to collect information from participants in a study making the data consistent independently on the source of data. The questions can represent different forms depending on the subject: open questions (the respondent answers with his/her own expressions – disadvantage – difficult to be classified), closed questions – the one or more versions of answers (multiple-choice) from among the given ones to be selected by the respondent.

# R

**Random sample** – the set of elements of equal probability for each one to be selected. For example the patients' selection to the clinical trial.

**Range** – the interval of values as appears in particular sample. The value of range is expressed by the difference between the maximum and minimum value in the sample.

**Record of information** – complete set of data (with unit definition) addressed to the respondent.

**Regression analysis** – the technique to recognize the characteristics (shape) and power of relation (association) between two variables. *See* linear regression.

**Regression Linear** – *See* linear regression.

   **Nonlinear** – *See* nonlinear regression.

**Rejection region** – the range of values of statistics above and below the critical values defined by the level of significance and number of degrees of freedom. *See* decision rules.

**Relative frequency** – proportion of values falling within the class interval versus the total number of observations. Usually expressed in percentage.

# S

**Sample size determination** – the critical issue for statistical analysis due to the reliability of the results received using statistical analysis which is specifically oriented on large-number analysis of populations. The main goal is to be able to spread the conclusions on the general population what is impossible for small size samples. The proper number of elements in the sample classifies the sample as representative one. The procedure allowing calculation of necessary number of elements is available for measurable and quantitative variables on the basis of pilot studies allowing estimation of the frequency of the event under consideration.

**Scatter-plot (Scatter-diagram)** – the graphical presentation of two measurable variables in the Cartesian coordinate system. Each point represents values of two variables (one determines the position on horizontal axis and other on the vertical axis) making possible the visual assessment of their mutual relationship.

**Screening studies** – investigations of the healthcare character aimed to recognize the high versus low probability of the given disorder (serious public health condition in population). The preclinical and early diagnosis, safer treatment, lowering the invasiveness of the procedures, reduction of mortality). The effect of such analysis is the wide introduction of mammography, blood tests to identify the specific antigens (cancer diseases), blood pressure as the symptoms for heart diseases. The screening tests are oriented on lowering costs, analysis of target population, etc.

**Significance level** – the desired level to define the critical region of particular test. Probability of rejecting a true null hypothesis.

**Simple linear regression** – the linear function assumed to represent the form of the relation between variable $x$ called as independent and the $y$ variable – the dependent one.

> **Estimation of parameters** – to treat the regression function as representative for experimental points (scatter diagram); the two parameters of linear regression function (slope and intercept) undergo the estimation verifying their significance.

**Simple random sample** – the basic sampling technique to choose by chance the elements of population to the sample. Each element of population has an equal probability of being chosen to be the element of the sample. The sampling is performed in form without the replacement what means, that each element can be chosen only once.

**Slope** – the parameter "a" present in linear function influencing the orientation of the line versus the coordinate system axes.

**Standard deviation** – measurements of the dispersion of values in the sample equal to the square root of variance.

**Standard normal distribution** – normal distribution with mean $\bar{x} = 0.0$ and standard deviation $s = 1.0$. *See* normal distribution.

**Standardization procedure** – transformation of any measurable variable into the universal form expressed by $Z$ variable (*See* $Z$ variable). Each $X$ value subtracted from mean value and divided by standard deviation transforms the set of "$X$" into the set of "$Z$" of mean value equal to 0 and standard deviation equal to 1.0.

**Statistical interference** – the technique by which the conclusion about a population on the basis of the information contained in a sample can be drawn from that population.

**Statistical methods** – set of methods oriented on collection, organization, summarization and analysis of data together with the procedures allowing drawing of inferences about a body of data when only a part of the data is observed.

**Statistical tables** – tables summarizing the critical values for number of degrees of freedom and assumed level of significance.

**Skewness** – the measure of the asymmetry of the probability distribution. The asymmetry can represent the left-hand skew when the maximum of function is moved toward low values of the variable, and (the) right-hand skew with the maximum moved toward higher values of the variable under consideration. Skewness of the distribution can be easily recognized by comparing three parameters of central tendency: left-handed $Mo > Me > \bar{x}$ ; for right-handed $\bar{x} > Me > Mo$.

**Standard deviation** – the measure of spread versus the mean value assumed to represent the central tendency position. The interval $\bar{x} \pm s$ covers 68% of the total area under the Gauss curve (the finding of the value from this interval is equal 68%), the interval $\bar{x} \pm 2s$ covers 95% of the total area under the Gauss curve and the interval $\bar{x} \pm 3s$ covers 99.7% of the total area under the Gauss function for normal distribution.

**Standard error** – the standard deviation of the sampling distribution of a statistics. For example – the standard error of the sample mean of $n$ observations is $s/\sqrt{n}$ .

**Statistical packages** – the Association for Survey Computing (ASC) website (www.asc.org.uk) listed over than 150 statistical packages a few years ago. Some of them have been developed for many years like SPSS (www.spss.com), SAS (www.sas.com), STATA (www.stata.com), S-Plus (www.insightful.com), Genstat (www.vsn-intl.com), Statistica (www.statsoft.com), NCSS (www.ncss.com), SYSTAT (www.systat.com). Some of them are specialized (for example – Genstat for molecular biology, SPSS for social sciences). All of them are possible to run on PC. All of them offer the "Help" tool with quite wide and precise theoretical explanation of the methods applied. What is very important – the import/export of data allowing communication with other packages is available in all of them.

**Stem-and-leaf plot** – one of the graphical presentation(s) of the set of data (similar to the histogram). Data is arranged by place value, the digits in the largest place form stem and the less important digits form leaves. The column on the left side (stem) gives the list of the third and second highest positions of the values (measurements of particular variable) and then the third position is given in form of row (leaves) attached to the appropriate position of the third and second position of the value.

**Student's test** – usually treated equivalently with T-test – the parametric test assessing the difference between mean values in two groups as negligibly small (null hypothesis) or significantly different (alternative hypothesis). The analysis takes into consideration the number of elements in each group (number of degrees of freedom), mean values in both groups and their variances. The assumption of normality distribution in each group shall be satisfied before the application of the T-test.

**Survival analysis** – methods for the analysis of time-to-event data, in particular survival time, although other endpoints are possible. The time range between (the) well defined starting point (appearance of particular symptoms) and (the) end-point (appearance of particular event – recurrence of symptoms).

**Survival curve** – *See* Kaplan-Meier plot.

# T

**The inference statistics** – techniques revealing the significance of differences or of relations between variables under consideration suggesting the search for possible mechanisms responsible for discovered relationships. The main goal of statistical analysis is to make possible the generalization (the conclusion generated on the basis of sample analysis to be generalized to the whole population) of the observed relations, what significantly depends on the quality of data collected and of the number of observations.

**T-test** – *See* the t-Student test.

**Two-sided test** – form to express the alternate hypothesis when no direction for the difference is specified. For example – two compared mean values satisfy the relation: $\bar{x}_A \neq \bar{x}_B$ without specification of the direction of this inequality. *See* one-sided test.

**Type error I** – the probability to reject the null hypothesis which is in reality true.

**Type error II** – the probability to accept the null hypothesis when in reality the alternate hypothesis is true.

# V

**Variability** – measure of spread – range, standard deviation, variance.

**Variable**

    **continuous** – *See* continuous variable,

    **dependent** – two events are in relation that the occurrence of one of them influences the probability the second one to occur – *See* independent variable,

    **discrete** – *See* discrete variable,

    **independent** – *See* independent variable,

    **quantitative (measurable)** – obtained as the result of measurements in the usual sense.

    **qualitative (descriptive)** – variable which is not capable of being measured like color, shape, profession, etc.

**Variance** – one of the forms to measure the dispersion of values in the sample or in the population equal to the square of the standard deviation.

**Variance estimation** *See* F-test.

# W

**Which test to use** – the selection of test depends on the: character of the variable (measurable or qualitative), number of samples under assessment, distribution character (normal or non-normal distribution).

**Wilcoxon rang sum test** – *See* Mann-Whitney rank sum test.

# Y

**y-intercept** – *See* intercept.

# Z

**Z-score** – the standardized value of an observation X calculated by subtracting the sample mean and dividing by sample standard deviation. In consequence the mean value of Z is equal 0.0. and standard deviation equal(s) to 1.0.

## Following manuals are recommended for further readings:

BIOSTATISTICS – A GUIDE TO DESIGN, ANALYSIS AND DISCOVERY
RONALD N. FORTHOFER. EUN SUL LEE AND MICHAEL HERNANDEZ, ELSEVIER, ACADEMIC PRESS, 2007
ENCYCLOPAEDIC COMPANION TO MEDICAL STATISTICS, EDITED BY BRIAN S. EVERITT AND CHRISTOPHER R. PALMER, 2005, HODDER ARNOLD
BIOSTATISTICS: A FOUNDATION FOR ANALYSIS IN THE HEALTH SCIENCES – WAYNE W. DANIEL, JOHN WILEY & SONS INC. 1999, SEVENTH EDITION.

# INDEX

# CONTENTS

TECHNICAL EDITORS
*Jadwiga Makowiec*
*Marta Janiszewska-Hanusiak*

Wydawnictwo Uniwersytetu Jagiellonskiego
Redakcja: ul. Michałowskiego 9/2, 31-126 Kraków
tel. 012-631-18-81, tel./fax 012-631-18-83